Unraveling the Cancer Puzzle: From Complexity to Fundamental Properties

Zaki

Contents

Chapter 1

Introduction

Historically, many breakthroughs in physics resulted from coarse graining of complex systems, focusing on their most fundamental properties and interactions. Often it is easier to incorporate second order effects later. These successes are a strong motivation to search for coarse grained descriptions of complex systems of interest. In the case of this thesis the system of interest is biological tissue in general and cancer specifically. The motivation for studying cancer hardly needs an introduction. It is globally the second leading cause of death and about one in six people die of cancer [1]. Most of the effort in cancer research has been from the biological and genetics point of view, where the disease is incredibly complicated. The fundamental problem is that cancer develops out of consecutive mutations of the genome of previously healthy cells, which are inherently random. This causes strong genetic differences between cancers of different patients and even large genetic heterogeneities within one tumour [2, 3, 4]. This means that progress from biological research, targeting specific cell features is often restricted to a certain type of cancer, such as hormone treatment for receptor-positive (oestrogen/progesterone/HER2) breast cancer patients [5]. Of cause, every improvement in treatment or diagnosis that helps to save lives is important, but the general pace of progress has been slow compared to the effort that was put into cancer research, mostly because of the biological fragmentation and complexity of the disease [6, 7, 8, 9].

In cases like these, where research has been stuck or at least seems suboptimal, orthogonal approaches stand a chance to make an impact and this is the direction of my thesis. Regardless of their genetic and molecular make-up, tumours and cancer cells have to develop the right physical properties to achieve physical processes like invasion and metastasis. It is a priori reasonable to assume that the ability of cells to be able to move inside tissues and leave it is connected with their ability to metastasise. The focus in this thesis lies on the emergent collective behaviour of tissues depending on their constituting cells. Until recently, physicists generally regarded tissues as fluids on long time scales, supported by observations of cell sorting [10, 11, 12], liquid-like droplet fusion [13, 14], wetting [15, 16, 17] and surface tension with viscous behaviour for long time scales [18, 19, 20]. This fluid behaviour is associated with the ability of cells to rearrange inside the tissue, but this way of thinking has been started to get challenged recently by observations of an arrest in cellular motion, especially in epithelial tissues, that has been classified as either glassy or jammed [21, 22, 23, 24, 25, 26]. There have been different approaches in theories to explain this behaviour, ranging from friction caused by adhesion [27], to density inspired by granular jamming [28], contact inhibition [29] and cell shape-dependent jamming [30, 31, 32]. Some of these theories have contradicting predictions, like an increasing adhesion leading to jamming in friction-driven theories and unjamming in shape-driven ones [27, 30], but most of them are consistent and might describe different facets of the system. Besides some evidence that cell shape [26] and cell density [21] are involved in the arrest of cellular motion in tissues, it is not clear which of these theories describe the most fundamental interaction, or if there are two distinct processes and how they are connected. The work in this thesis provides new insights regarding this question. I provide strong evidence that there is a shape-dependent jamming transition in two and three-dimensional confluent tissue and show that additional effects of cell number density are consistent with a reduced internal velocity of cells. I show that this physics is crucial to cancer research by detecting both arrested and fluid-like regions in primary human tumour pieces. Additionally, I demonstrate that a biological process that is typical for cancer progression causes an unjamming transition in cancer spheroids. This unjamming transition accompanied by a prominent loss of cohesion and a reduced volume fraction of cells, showing that cell jamming requires a high volume fraction [33].

The reason this cell jamming transition, as it has been mostly called, appears to be relevant for cancer progression, is that about 80 percent of cancers are carcinomas [9] developing out of epithelial tissues. These epithelial tissues are the standard example of jammed systems in the current literature of cell jamming. One of the hallmarks of cancer progression is the epithelial-mesenchymal transition [34], which is strongly connected to the metastatic ability of tumours, even though it is neither necessary nor sufficient for malignant behaviour [35, 36, 37, 38, 39]. It is a natural hypothesis, that this transition to a mesenchymal phenotype is connected to an unjamming transition of the tissue. Despite the importance of this hypothesis, it had not been confirmed until the work in this thesis. Part of my work was a cooperation with the group of Prof. Friedl to tackle this question. His group prepared 4T1 cells with stably down regulated E-cadherin, an adhesion molecule connected with multiple pathways whos down regulation is central to the epithelial-mesenchymal transition [40, 41, 38, 42]. The 4T1 cancer cell line is categorised by biologists as malignant and metastatic, but still retains many epithelial characteristics [43, 44]. Using cell tracking of spheroids at an interface expanding into collagen networks, I show that the down regulation switches the tissue behaviour from a collectively, persistent moving phenotype which has a low relative cell motion of close by cells to an uncoordinated, diffusive-like cell motion. This shows that the untreated 4T1 are at least close to a jamming transition and the motion of cells is impaired by their neighbours, while the E-cadherin down regulated phenotype switches to an individual cell motion not strongly influenced by neighbouring cells. This fluidisation is consistent between *in vitro* experiments and *in vivo* experiments in mice. Using a custom cell segmentation of fixated slices I was able to show that the reduction in E-cadherin leads to an individualisation of cells within the spheroid. Even if they are confined by a dense collagen matrix, there are cell free holes in the E-cadherin down regulated spheroids, which is not true for the untreated 4T1 spheroids. The constituting cells are more elongated and less densely packed in the E-cadherin down regulated spheroids. E-cadherin down regulated 4T1 cells were able to invade 2 mg/ml dense collagen networks as individual cells, in contrast to their untreated brethren, but were not able to achieve this in denser 6 mg/ml networks.

Furthermore, I could show that primary human tumour pieces contain fluid as well as arrested regions. These tumours pieces were densely-packed near volume fraction one. In order to investigate these different states in three-dimensional tissues, I used reproducible spheroids of cancer cell lines. I demonstrated different collective states of tissue behaviour in macroscopic rheological behaviour as well as microscopic cellular movement between epithelial-like MCF-10A cells and mesenchymal-like MDA-MB-436 cells [45], whose spheroids were also close to volume fraction one. For the first time in studies of three-dimensional tissues, I was able to connect the state of motility in the tissue with the cell shapes of the constituting cells using a custom self-developed 3D cell segmentation on fixated 3D stacks of confocal fluorescence images. Cells in the core of MCF-10A spheroids were significantly rounder and had a higher number density than the cells of MDA-MB-436 spheroids, correlating with theories of shape-dependent jamming as well as theories of density dependent jamming [32, 46, 47]. Very interestingly, I found a strong correlation between the shape of cells and their nuclei in the fixed spheroids, which means that there is also a correlation between cell jamming and the nucleus shape in this system, similar to individual cell movements in confining extracellular matrix [48, 49, 50]. I could confirm this behaviour in the primary tumour pieces, where the fluidly moving areas have cells with more elongated nuclei than the cells in arrested regions. This indicates that the nucleus deformations required for cell rearrangements contribute the energy barriers for cell rearrangements, since a higher energy would be required to sufficiently deform round nuclei. Therefore, my data suggests a biophysical underpinning of the histological prognostic marker of nuclei pleomorphism [51, 52].

With these results demonstrating the importance of the cellular jamming transition, the question what the main underlying cause of cellular jamming is becomes more pressing. One of the reasons, that there is no consensus regarding this question, is that the experimental evidence is only based on correlations between the properties of different ensembles and multiple of these properties are reported to be relevant in different publications [21, 26, 27, 53]. I improve on this approach by fine tuning a cell tracking algorithm that allows me to use measures of cell rearrangements such as the magnitude of non-affine displacement D^2_{min} that have a drastically higher spatial and temporal resolution than the measures that are used by particle image velocity analysis. I studied epithelial-like MCF-10A layers while the layers become denser through cell proliferation and transition into an arrested state. The temporal resolution allows me to study the transition process. I find no evidence for a first order state- or phase transition since the observed changes were smooth. The spatial resolution allows me study the dependency of the rearrangement speed of cells on the structural properties of their environment. This approach directly confirms that the local structural properties of the neighbouring cells have a strong influence of the relative motion of cells in densely-packed epithelial layers, experimentally justifying the description of caging that is often used. Both the mean cell shape of the neighbourhood as well as the respective mean cell number density have a strong influence on the local rearrangement dynamics. The rearrangement dynamic measured by the magnitude of non-affine displacement D^2_{min} can be rescaled with the difference of the mean shape of the cells neighbourhood to the critical cell shape index $p^* \approx 3.81$ of the vertex models of cell jamming [30]. This means that the difference of this mean cell shape to the critical cell shape index can be understood as a control parameter of the ability of cells to rearrange, similar to critical scaling behaviour near a phase transition. Therefore, this is profound evidence for a shape-dependent jamming transition. The additional effect of increasing number density is consistent with a slow down of the intrinsic cell velocity, which alone would only increase the viscosity of the fluid tissue and not jam it.

Overall, the work of this thesis proves that tumours can behave fluidly, solidly or, consistent with known biological tumour heterogeneity, both fluidly and solidly in different regions. These dynamical changes potentially have a large impact on the ability of tumours to metastasise, since they already show a drastically different invasion behaviour concerning the extracellular matrix [33]. Importantly, the dynamic behaviour of the tissue is reflected in its structure, providing strong motivation for the hypothesis that these structural features, observed in histological slides of tumours, could provide good prognostic markers for cancer development. Thereby, my thesis has inspired a collaboration of the group of my supervisor Prof. Käs with the pathologist Prof. Niendorf studying this possibility.

Chapter 2

Background

In this chapter I will discuss the background information necessary to understand this thesis. The scope of topics ranges from cell and cancer biology to tissue mechanics and the physics of glass and jamming transitions. For this reason, I will only give a short overview about the general topics and concentrate on the information that are particularly important regarding this thesis.

2.1 Basics of tumour biophysics

2.1.1 Cell biology

I will also focus on the features of cells necessary for cell motility in dense tissues. This section is adapted mostly from Alberts et al., Lodish et al. and Pollard et al. [54, 55, 56].

The basic building blocks of human tissue are eukaryotic cells. A sketch of the components of an eukaryotic cell, based on a fibroblast interacting with the extracellular matrix is shown in figure 2.1 reprinted from the textbook of Alberts et al. [54].

The largest structure in the cell is its nucleus, containing the genetic information of the cell necessary to build its proteins. It is enveloped by a lamin meshwork stabilising the nucleus and connecting it with the other components of the cytoskeleton. In typical mammalian cells, the nucleus inhabits roughly 10 percent of the cell volume, but more in cancer cells [57]. The nucleus does not actively deform during cell movement,

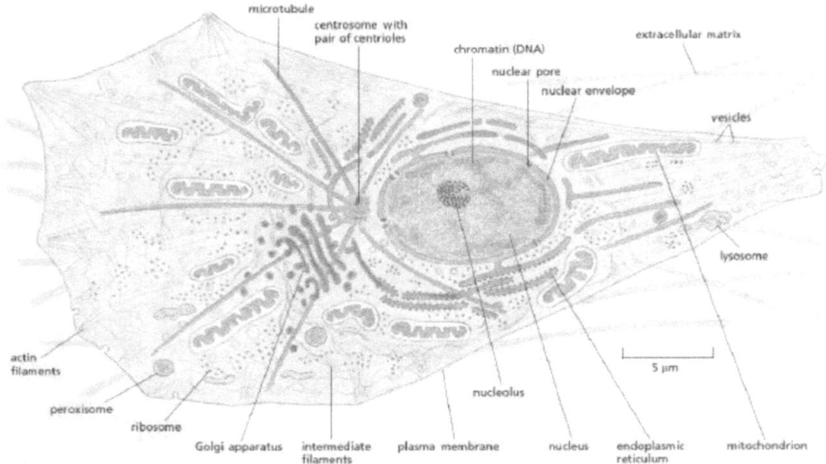

Figure 2.1: Schematic representation of a cell and its components. The basis of this particular drawing is a fibroblast cell. Reproduced from [54] under the terms of the Creative Commons CC BY-NC license. Copyright 2015, Yale Journal of Biology and Medicine.

in contrast to the cytoskeleton, and is therefore an object that passively resists cell motion through dense environments. It has been reported that the nucleus stiffness and deformation is correlated with ability of cell to move through narrow channels and dense extracellular matrix, where the movement sometimes even ruptures the nuclei, but this connection has not yet been shown for cell movement through dense tissue [48, 49, 50, 58, 59, 60, 61].

Cells are compartmentalised by the plasma membrane and thereby build the smallest living unit of tissues. The central part of the plasma membrane, or cell membrane, is a lipid bilayer that can self-assemble driven by entropic principles of its amphiphilic lipid components. Judging by molecular weight, only about 50 percent of the plasma membrane is build up by lipids and the other half consists of cholesterol and proteins. The cell membrane is semi-permeable and contains a plethora of different functional proteins, allowing the cell to control the amount of water, ions and small molecules that cross its boundary. Signalling proteins located in the cell membrane allow for communication with the outside, for example, by providing an accessible receptor for binding of hormones that trigger a signalling cascade on the inside of the cell.

Adhesion molecules are especially relevant for this thesis. They are located in the plasma membrane and can be connected to the cytoskeleton on the inside of the cell and different parts of the environment on the outside of the cell, like other cells or components of the extracellular matrix. The dissociation equilibrium constants of adhesion bounds are in the range of 1 to $100\,\mu$mol, which is low compared to other specific protein interactions, leading to dissociations times faster than one second for the binding [54]. This allows for the movement of cells, as there are repeated short time intervals between bindings, where the cells can rearrange and the stronger forces can break the bond. There are five major families of adhesion molecules: immunoglobulin–cell adhesion molecules, cadherins, selectins, mucins, that foster mainly cell-cell adhesions and integrins that are mainly bind to proteins of the extracellular matrix, but also other cells on some occasions [56]. Selectins and mucins mainly occur in white blood cells and endothelial cells, that are not the focus of this thesis, even though inflammation by white blood cells is strongly suspected as a tumour promoter [62]. The cell type that is most intersting regarding this thesis are epithelial cells, since malignant carcinomas develop out of them and this change is connected to a changed motility behaviour. For these epithelial cells, cadherins are the most typical family of adhesion molecules, especially E-cadherin and the desmosomal cadherins. Both of them exhibit homophilic interactions, binding to the same receptor in other cells. This favours strong binding of epithelial cells among each other over other cell types. Both of these adhesion molecules tend to cluster together forming adherens junctions and desmosomes between cells respectively. These clusters stabilise the adhesion more than individual molecules, since individual bindings are weak and short, but there are always other molecules connected when one is disrupted. E-cadherin is connected to the actin cytoskeleton on the inside of cells, while desmosomes are connected to keratin. E-cadherin is also involved in signaling processes inside the cell. For example, it has been shown that E-cadherin bounds reduce the actomyosin contractility along a cell-cell contact interface [63, 64, 65].

The last cell machinery that is of essential importance for the discussion of collective effects and cell motility is the cytoskeleton. Besides the direct involvement of some cytoskeleton structure on the cellular motility, it does modulate the stiffness of cells, which is important for movement in dense tissues, as stiffer cells are harder to push away. The main families of components are actin, intermediate filaments, and microtubules. All of them consist of smaller units like monomers or dimers, polymerises into chains of these called filaments, and then build up larger structures like networks, bundles or fibres.

Microtubles are most known for being involved in the cell division. In non-dividing cells they are orginised in a star-like structure from the microtubule-organising center. They have a plus and minus end, allowing motor proteins to transport organelles and vesicles on them in a directed fashion, thus providing a basis for the spatial organization in the cell. Since they are not central to the thesis, I will concentrate on actin and intermediate filaments.

The building block of actin structures are monomers of globular, so-called G-actin, that build up a helix conformation of two chains in one actin filament, called F-actin. In this thesis, I often use actin as a synonym for F-actin. These structures have a polarization plus and minus end, whereby the energy-consuming polymerization occurs mainly on the plus end. There are many different proteins inside the cell, that can influence the polymerisation and cross-linking of actin, controlling the structure and dynamics of the actin cytoskeleton. Actin is present in multiple kinds of structures in the cell. There is a dense network of actin directly under the plasma membrane connected to it that has an anchoring and stabilising function. Actin is present as a network in lamellipodia and in form of bundles in filopodia pushing the leading edge of the cell forward with polymerization at the plus end during crawling type cell movement. In epithelial cells actin bundles also occur in form of a circumferential belt under the plasma membrane connecting adherence junctions. These are partly cross-linked by myosin II motor proteins, that are able to exert forces to contract these rings, contributing to the contractile character and round cell shapes in the plane of epithelial tissue. Similar bundle structures exist between focal adhesions formed by integrins binding to the substrate or dense extracellular matrix. These bundles are called stress fibers and are cross linked by α-actinin and also associated with myosin II motor proteins. It is clear, that these stress fibres can exert contractile force between the focal adhesions, suggesting a role in cell migration, but their precise role in cell motility is not clear, as many cell types can move in many situations without stress fibres [66, 67, 68].

The main types of intermediated filaments are lamins, keratins, vimentin, desmin and neurofilaments. Intermediate filaments are not associated with motor proteins and cell movement in contrast to other cytoskeletal filaments. They play a role in the stabilisation of cells and the mediating adhesion. Lamins are located around nuclei, as described before. Desmins are mainly located in muscle cells and neurofilaments are mainly located in neurons, which are both not the focus of this work. On the other hand, there are keratins, which are typical for epithelial cells, whereby each type of epithelium expresses a characteristic combination of 20 acidic and basic cytokeratins.

Keratins are like actin commonly associated with the plasma membrane and are connected with desmosomes and hemidesmosomes that connect the cell to other cells and the extracellular matrix or substrate respectively. There are proteins such as plectin that crosslink cytokeratin and vimentin and also connect it to other filaments of the cytoskeleton like actin and microtubles.

From a physical perspective microtubles are the stiffest molecules, but tend to buckle under compressive stress [69]. However, they might be more impactful *in vivo* due to lateral support by other parts of the cytoskeleton [70, 71]. The actin cytoskeleton might be the main contributor for cell stiffness regarding small deformations, while the intermediated filaments are more durable for larger deformations that break other filaments [72, 73, 74, 75].

As mentioned above, the cellular process most relevant to this thesis is migration. There are different kinds of cell movement possible. One of them is called blebbing motion, whereby the actin cortex under the plasma membrane ruptures locally and leading to an inflation of the plasma membrane at this location due to the internal pressure of the cell [76, 77, 78]. The swelling of these blebs stops, when a new cortex is formed under the expanded plasma membrane [79, 80]. These protrusions can allow cells to establish a hold through narrow gaps in the extracellular matrix [81]. However, this mode of motility relies on the internal cell pressure to be higher than the external pressure, which is not necessary true in dense tissues, where the bleb would have to expand against the other cells. Combined with the fact that this mode of motility has not been observed in dense two- or three-dimensional tissue renders it of low importance for this thesis.

In the more widespread form of motion, often called crawling motion, protrusions are generated by actin polymerisation at the leading edge of cells. In case of actin forming networks, these are called lamellipodia and for bundles filopodia, while the collective term is pseudopodia. As mentioned earlier, actin has one end that polimerises about ten times faster than the other end. Near such a leading edge, whenever the plasma membranes fluctuate away from the end of the actin structure, new actin monomers have the chance to attach and push the leading edge forward in a treadmill-like fashion. Then, this protrusion builds up adhesive bonds, while the adhesive connections in the rear end of the cells are disengaged. Meanwhile, the cell body is moved by contractile forces. In lamellipodia, contractile forces, together with the continued proliferation at the front of the actin network, cause an effect called retrograde flow. This term describes the actin network near the leading edge being pushed back over time, which causes a traction force. The contractile forces are caused by myosin II motors interacting with actin structures in the cell, which are the cortex, the network at the leading edge and potentially stress fibres.

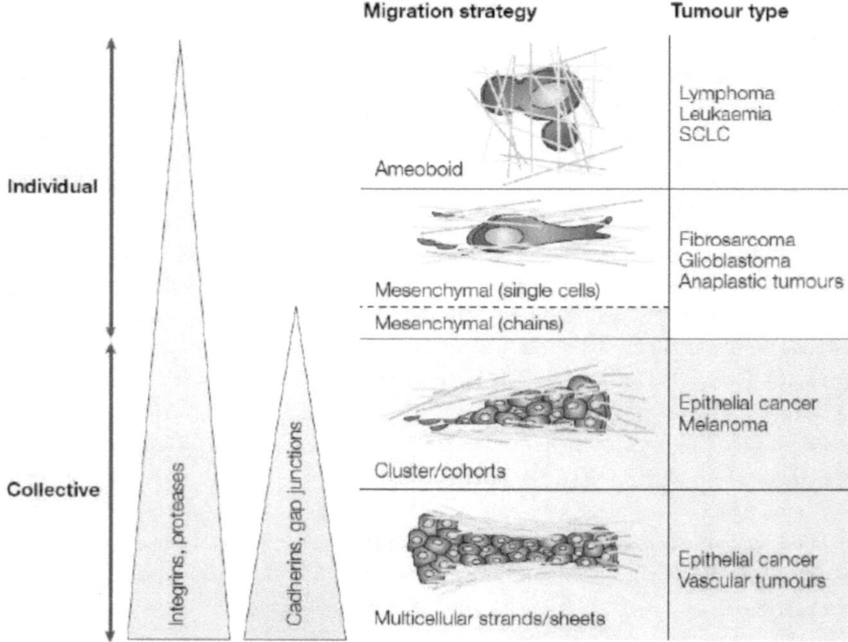

Figure 2.2: Types of cell motility connected to cancer invasion. Collectivity of motion and amount of adhesion proteins matrix metalloproteinases are indicated on the left. In the middle, sketches and names or migration modes are shown. On the right side tumour types, that typically use the respective migration modes are listed. Reprinted from [82]. Copyright ©2003 Springer Nature, license number 4997660428186.

A characterization of different migration strategies connected to cancer invasion is shown in figure 2.2 reprinted from Friedl et al [82]. Ameoboidly behaving cells can both employ blebbing and and crawling motion, depending on their excact make up and environment [83]. Their crawling motion is characterised by a lack of focal adhesions and stress fibres, indicating a comparably low contractile behaviour. Contrary, mesenchymal motion is typically a type of crawling motion that often contains focal adhesion and stress fibres. [84]

Besides these types of individual cell motion, there are types and environment where cells move collectivity. This is most typical for epithelial cells during wound healing [85, 86, 87], but it is also typical for tumours that develop out of epithelial tissue [82, 88, 89]. This behaviour is connected to a high amount of adhesion, particularly from E-cadherin and adhesion junction. In the extracellular matrix, collectively moving cancer cells often up-regulate matrix metalloproteinases to degrade the extracellular matrix in order to have space to move [90, 91, 92, 93]. Collective cellular movement has been connected with cell jamming [94]. This will be discussed further in 2.2.2 and throughout this thesis. There is also the fact, that the tumour environment can create a path of least resistance, leading the cells to move in the same region, which has been described as collective motion by biologists [95, 96, 97, 98, 89, 99, 100]. One of the results, presented later in this thesis, is that this confinement by the environment does not lead to the correlated and cohesive motion, that biophysicists would call collective motion. Instead this motion is correlated with the cell properties.

Cancer cells can transition between these different kind of motions [82, 84, 101, 102]. I will describe the transition from the epithelial to the mesenchymal phenotype in more detail in the next chapter, because one of the main findings of this thesis is the switch from a caged, collective behaviour to a fluid non-cohesive motility caused by the down regulation of E-cadherin, which is one of the typical features of this the epithelial-mesenchymal transition.

2.1.2 Cancer development

From the biological point of view, cancer is a very complicated disease, because it arises out of a series of random mutations of previously healthy cells. This makes the exact properties of each individual tumour, hard to predict and treat. Additionally, cancers developing out of different types of cells often keep some of their characteristics making the term cancer more of a collective term for different phenomena. For example there are sarcomas that develop from mesenchymal cells like fibroblasts, lymphomas developing out of lymphocytes, melanomas arising out of pigment cells in the skin and carcinomas that mutate from epithelial cells. There have been over 200 biologically different types of cancer found, which impedes the development of treatments based in their molecular profile [103]. Nevertheless, there are shared properties of different cancers summarised as hallmarks in the classic reviews of Hanahan and Weinberg [104, 34]. An overview of these hallmarks, reprinted from there 2011 review, is shown in figure 2.3. [34]

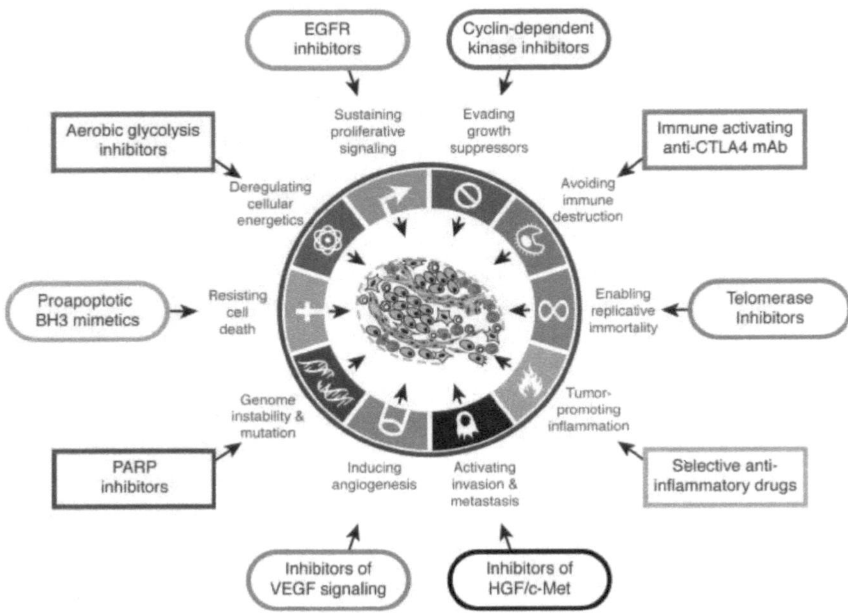

Figure 2.3: Hallmarks of cancer according to the classic review of Hanahan and Weinberg. The inner ring shows the typical shared properties of cancers. The outer ring shows molecular changes connected to these properties. Reprinted from [34]. Copyright ©2011 Elsevier, license number 4997670688338

The most basic changes of cancer cells at the start of cancer development are the ability to divide indefinitely and a resistance to apoptosis triggers. Connected to that is the production of their own growth signals and the insensitivity to growth suppressors. All of these chances are accomplished by genetic and epigenetic alterations inside the cancer cells. Another hallmark in this vain is the observed genome instability and genetic heterogeneity of tumours. Additionally, many of the other changes are also connected to such mutations, leading cancer to be seen as a genetic disease and research focusing in this direction [105, 106, 103]. However, as described earlier, there is an immense amount of complexity and diversity in cancer, which makes it unlikely that a therapy targeting a single gene can be effective against a large fraction of tumours [107, 108]. Consequently, there have been suggestions, for example by Sonnenschein and Soto, to shift the current paradigm away from genetics to a tissue-level disease [106]. The approach of this thesis fits well to this hypothesis. Returning the focus back to the shared properties of cancer summarised as hallmarks, cancer cells need a lot of energy and nutrients to allow their increased proliferation. This manifests in alterations of the metabolism of the cancer cells and an initiation of angiogensis in the tumour. Additionally, cancers develop features to avoid the immune system and induce inflammation, which promotes tumour development [109, 110].

The last hallmark of cancer described by Hanahan and Weinberg, that I did not mention yet, is the activation of tumour invasion and metastasis. Metastasis is the cause of at least two-thirds of cancer deaths [112]. An improvement in understanding the involved processes can therefore lead to strong improvements in diagnosis and treatment of cancer. I will concentrate on the case of carcinoma, developing out of internal epithelial tissue. A schematic showing the steps required for metastasis, reprinted from Bacac and Stamenkovic, is shown in figure 2.4 [111]. Before the invasion of the surrounding environment can begin, the tumour has to develop out of a carcinoma in situ into an invasive phenotype and degrade the basement membrane. This requires already most of the hallmarks of cancer discussed above and describes the difference between benign and malignant tumours. The microenvironment of tumours is often directly or indirectly adjusted by the tumour, for example by inflammation, cancer associated fibroblasts and tumour associated macrophages [113, 114, 115]. This is important for tumour growth, but of course might also influence the potential cancer invasion. The ability to express matrix metalloproteinases, degrading extracellular matrix proteins is also often up-regulated in malignant cancer [90, 91, 92, 93]. The different migration strategies of cancer cells in the extracellular matrix have already been introduced in the previous chapter. From the side of cellular mechanics, the most prominent change connected to the matrix invasion is the epithelial-mesenchymal transition, which will be discussed in more detail in the next paragraph [37]. The next step required for distant metastasis is the intravasion of blood or lymph vessels by these cancer cells. The prerequisite for this process is either the angiogensis in the primary tumour or the reaching of blood or lymph vessels by tumour growth or invasion. Similar to matrix invasion, tumour associated cells like fibroblasts or macrophages can increase the ability of cancer cells to conduct the intravasion [116]. Cancer cells that have undergone an epithelial-mesenchymal transition have a higher ability to overcome the

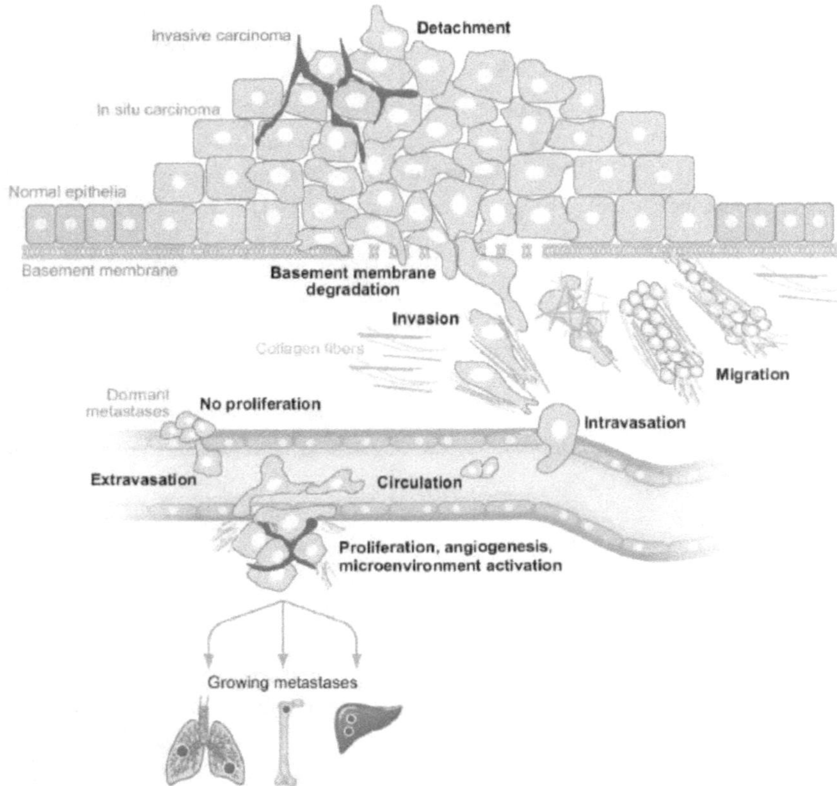

Figure 2.4: Schematic of the steps of cancer metastasis. The development of a carcinoma in situ is followed by a transformation into an invasive phenotype and the degradation of the basement membrane. The invasion of the extracellular matrix, is followed by the intravasion of blood or lymph vessels. A distant metastasis requires survival in the vessel, extravasation at the side and a continued survival and proliferation of the cancer cells at this side. The figure is reprinted from [111] with permission from Annual Reviews, Inc. (Order licence ID 1093640-1).

endothelium of blood vessels [117]. In the blood and lymph vessels, cancer cells are exposed to an increased amount of immune cells rendering their adaptation in deceiving the immune system is of great importance for survival [118]. Early scientific results show that clusters of circulating tumour cells are more resilient regarding cancer cells and more likely to cause metastasis [119, 120, 118]. The metastasis requires both the ability to leave the blood vessel, called extravasation, and the ability to survive and proliferate in the new environment. Interestingly, a mesenchymal phenotype is not of advantage for extravasation, which is even connected to a mesenchymal-epithelial transition [117]. There are different cellular subpopulations differently well adapted to the different potential metastatic sites in the body, increasing the importance of tumour heterogeneity for metastasis [121, 122, 123].

A reoccurring theme in the background part is the epithelial-mesenchymal transition, which is connected to many of the processes during cancer metastasis. This transition also happens in healthy bodies during embryogenesis and tissue regeneration, where the resulting mesenchymal-like cells can secrete proteins of the extracellular matrix [38]. These existing pathways for cellular change get co-opted during cancer development. Interestingly, the epithelial-mesenchymal transition during tissue regeneration is accompanied by inflammation and potentially fibrosis, which are also known tumour promoters [38, 124, 125]. In cancer progression, inflammation is reported to induce the epithelial-mesenchymal transition and vice versa [126, 127]. The molecular causes of the epithelial-mesenchymal transition are extremely complex: "In the case of many carcinomas, EMT-inducing signals emanating from the tumor-associated stroma, notably HGF, EGF, PDGF, and TGF-β, appear to be responsible for the induction or functional activation in cancer cells of a series of EMT-inducing transcription factors, notably Snail, Slug, zinc finger E-box binding homeobox 1 (ZEB1), Twist, Goosecoid, and FOXC2 [35, 128, 129, 130, 131, 132]"[38]. Other mediators include Notch, Wnt and hypoxia [133, 134, 135]. There is also the possibility of a partial epithelial-mesenchymal transition, rendering the situation more complex [136, 137].

Figure 2.5 displays a sketch showing the molecular changes during the epithelial-mesenchymal transition, reprinted from [38]. From a physical perspective, the most important changes shown are the switching of E-cadherin and cytokeratins to N-cadherin and vimentin respectively. The switch away from E-cadherin reduces the cell-cell adhesion by impeding the possibility of cells to form adherens junctions and tight junctions, which is not balanced out by N-cadherin proteins [138, 41, 101, 135]. The disappearance of cytokeratins disrupts desmosomes, additionally decreasing cell-cell adhesion

[101, 139, 135]. Besides the change in adhesion, there occurs a drastic reorganisation of the cytoskeleton during the epithelial-mesenchymal transition [140, 141, 142]. This reduces active force transmission, coordination across multiple cell bodies, coordination of actomyosin contractility and multicellular polarity [143, 144, 145, 146]. The reorganisation of the actin cytoskeleton increases the ability of the cells to generate pseudopodia, that are used in cell motility [140, 145]. Additionally, the switch from cytokeratin to vimentin increases the motility of cells [147, 148, 145].

The precise influence of the epithelial-mesenchymal transition on cancer metastasis is complex and not completely understood [149]. There is a lot of evidence, that the epithelial-mesenchymal transition can promote metastasis in certain cases, but it is not required and investigations on metastatic outcome based on the status of the epithelial-mesenchymal transition had varying results [35, 150, 138, 151, 152, 153, 154, 149, 100, 155]. The epithelial-mesenchymal transition can certainly promote invasion in the local extracellular matrix and intravasion into blood vessels, but the distant metastatic tumour typically have epithelial characteristics [40, 151, 156]. There are several potential routes to metastasis, regarding the epithelial-mesenchymal transition and it is currently not clear, which of those occur to what extend and under which circumstances. The first possibility is that cancer cells undergo an epithelial-mesenchymal transition to migrate to a distant organ, followed by the reverse mesenchymal-epithelial transition to adapt to the organ [117, 156]. The second possibility is that the tumour heterogenity leads to both mesenchymal-like as well as epithelial-like cancer cells, which would allow the mesenchymal-like cells to 'pave the way' and help the epithelial-like to reach distant regions, where they are better equipped to survive [157, 158, 159, 116, 160]. Another

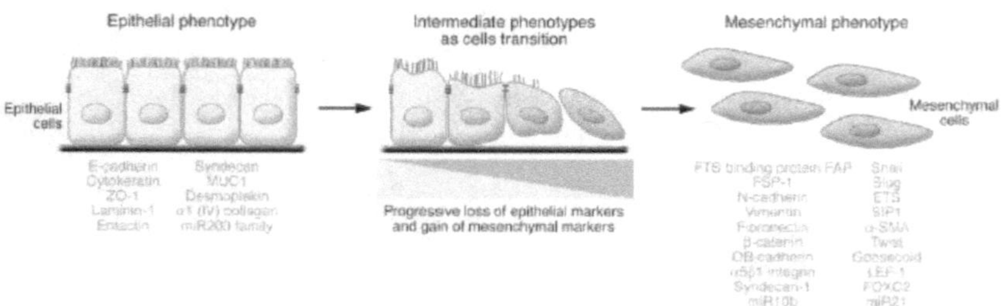

Figure 2.5: Molecular changes during the epithelial-mesenchymal transition. Reprinted from [38] with permission from the American Society for Clinical Investigation (Order licence ID 1093650-1).

possibility is that the truly dangerous phenotype is the one of a partially undergone epithelial-mesenchymal transition, because it is in a metastable state and the cells are able to switch phenotypes as they need, either directly by undergoing parts of the transition or evolutionary as survival of the fittest [136, 137, 161, 162]. Of course there is also the possibilty, that multiple potential pathways to metastasis exist and a metastasis occurs when the requirements for one of them are fulfilled. Even though there is already a large amount of research regarding the epithelial-mesenchymal transition, it is clear that more research is needed to unravel this complexity. The work presented in thesis contributes by showing that the down regulation of E-cadherin, the major hallmark of the epithelial-mesenchymal transition, causes an unjamming transition of the tissue (see chapter 4.2).

2.2 Tissue mechanics

In this chapter, I will present the basis of tissue mechanics necessary to understand this thesis. I will focus on the jamming transition in biological tissues. This chapter is loosely based on recent reviews of this topic by Oswald et al. and Park et al. [163, 164].

2.2.1 Fluid-like tissue dynamics

Biophysicists have treated tissues as viscoelastic material for a long time. The basic assumption was, that elastic solid-like behaviour on short time scales and viscous fluid-like behaviour on long time scales represent the properties of tissues well. An early example of this assumption of viscous fluid-like behaviour on long time scales is the pioneering differential adhesion hypothesis that was developed by Malcolm Steinberg in the nineteen-sixties [10, 165]. It was observed, that different cell populations sort themselves reliably into inner spheres and outer shells. This behaviour was explained by the hypothesis, that the cells behave like an immiscible liquid and demix based on their individual tissue surface tension, which arises from differences in adhesion. The resulting cell sorting is consistent with many different cell types, that were experimentally studied [10, 11, 19, 166, 12]. The segregation that occurs in these systems requires the ability of cells to rearrange inside the tissue. In a solid-like system the cells would have to stay in or near their original neighbourhood and the system would depend on the initial conditions. There have been multiple adjusted differential adhesion hypotheses

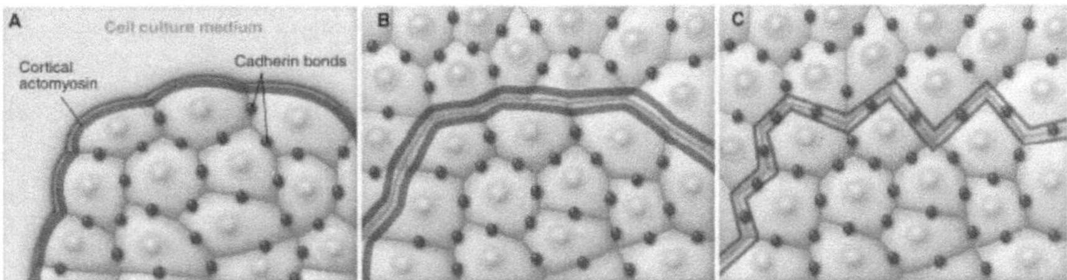

Figure 2.6: Sketch explaining the extended differential adhesion hypothesis. Cadherin bounds are indicated as red dots and a larger than average amount of the cortical actomyosin is indicated in green, whereby the line thickness expresses the amount of additional actomyosin corresponding to the generated tension. From [65]. Reprinted with permission from AAAS.

proposed that use cell contractility rather than adhesion [167], or both cell contractility and adhesion [167] or a co-regulated system of cadherin mediated adhesion and cortical tension [168, 65]. A sketch illustrating the last mentioned hypothesis is shown in figure 2.6. It is based on the finding that the measured tissue surface is orders of magnitude larger than it should be if it was just caused by the adhesion molecules and the finding that E-cadherin mediated adhesion decreases the actomyosin contractility along an interface connected via cadherin bonds [169, 63, 64, 168, 65]. The decreased contractility on the inside of cell clusters of the same cell leads to an effective tension on the interface between different cell types, explaining the tissue surface tension responsible for demixing [65]. Despite the differences, all these theories assume the ability of cells to rearrange themselves inside the tissue and therefore a fluid-like tissue behaviour on long time scales. This assumption has not been challenged until recently [170, 171].

Multiple experimental methods to measure the viscous fluid-like behaviour that many tissues exhibit are shown in figure 2.7, as composed by [163]. The upper line of images, labelled A, shows cell segregation experiments similar to the experiments described in the previous paragraph. These specific segregation experiments are especially interesting regarding this thesis, because they do not follow any of the theories of differential adhesion described above [170]. I will explain this further in the chapter about solid-like behaviour. The second row of images, labelled B, shows the fusion of cell spheroids build up by cardiac cushion tissue. The behaviour of these cellular spheroids resembles those of liquid droplets, where the surface tension drives the fusion and is impeded by the viscosity of the material [14]. Similar dynamic behaviour in accordance to viscous

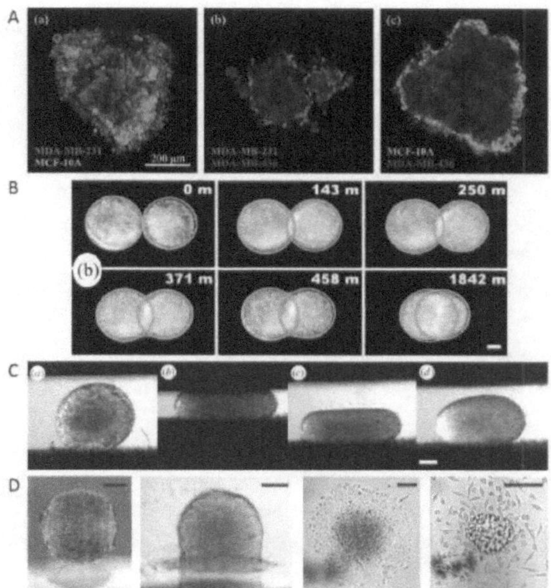

Figure 2.7: Compilation of methods measuring the viscous response of spheroids or tissues, originally arranged by Oswald et al. [163]. ©IOP Publishing Ltd and Deutsche Physikalische Gesellschaft. CC BY 3.0. **A**, Demixing of different breast cell lines in three-dimensional spheroids. Reproduced from [170]. ©IOP Publishing Ltd and Deutsche Physikalische Gesellschaft. CC BY 3.0. **B**, Fusion experiments of spherical aggregates build up by cardiac cushion tissue. Reprinted from [14] with permission from APS. ©2012 by the American Physical Society. **C**, Tissue surface tensiometer measurement by compression and relaxation of embryonic tissue. Reprinted from [25]. ©2013 The Author(s) Published by the Royal Society. All rights reserved. (Order licence ID 1093910-1) **D**, Process of wetting of a cell spheroid on a glass surface. The left images show the initial state and a partial wetting. The right images show the final state and a transition to a two-dimensional gas-like behaviour. These images were originally compiled in the review [17]. Reprinted with permission from AAAS. The two left are from [16]. Reprinted with permission from Royal Society of Chemistry (Order licence ID 1093918-1). The two right images are from [15]. Reprinted with permission from AAAS.

hydrodynamics is reported for multiple embryonic tissues [172, 13, 173]. The tissue surface tension, that has been mentioned both in the explanation for cell segregation and spheroid fusion and can be measured with a tissue surface tensiometer [174] as shown in the images labelled as C in figure 2.7 which have been reprinted from [25]. This has been done mostly for embryonic tissue, which typically displays an elastic response for short time scales and a viscous response on long time scales [19, 18, 20]. Another feature of fluid-like tissue behaviour is wetting. This is shown in the bottom row of images in figure 2.7 [15, 16, 17]. The degree of wetting from non-wetting, partial wetting to complete wetting is dependent on the ratio between cell-cell adhesion and cell-substrate adhesion [15, 16, 17]. If the cell-substrate adhesion is low enough cells form spheroids by nucleation and growth, by a process called de-wetting [175, 176].

2.2.2 Solid-like tissue dynamics

It is intuitively clear, that not all tissues can behave fluid-like on a long time scale, since the overall behaviour of living bodies is solid on long time scale. Theoretically, this solid-like behaviour could be maintained by active processes, that compensate the fluid processes, but this would be complex to adjust and energetically inefficient for the body. The hypothesis, that solid-like tissues exist is therefore a priori persuasive. Fluid-like behaviour requires the possibility of cells to rearrange in the tissue. In situations, where the tissue is confluent or close to confluent, these rearrangements requires the motion or deformation of neighbouring cells. It is therefore possible to imagine a state where this motion or deformation requires more energy than the cell that tries to move can exhibit, leading to a caging of the cell by its neighbours, in analogy to the concept of jamming of colloids. The collective arrest in motion within tissues has usually been called cellular jamming, because one of the early influential theory papers coined its finding a jamming transition, since it did not include cell motility [30]. This term permeated the literature, since it is instructive, which is a large advantage in interdisciplinary research. Thus, I will mostly use the terminology of jamming throughout this thesis, even though the term glass-like behaviour would be more correct from a physicists point of view, because cells have a non-vanishing activity [177].

The first experiments indicating effects of this nature are illustrated in figure 2.8. In 2011 Angelini et al. reported a slow down of velocity in epithelial monolayers, that they characterised as glass-like [21]. They reported dynamic heterogeneities, similar to

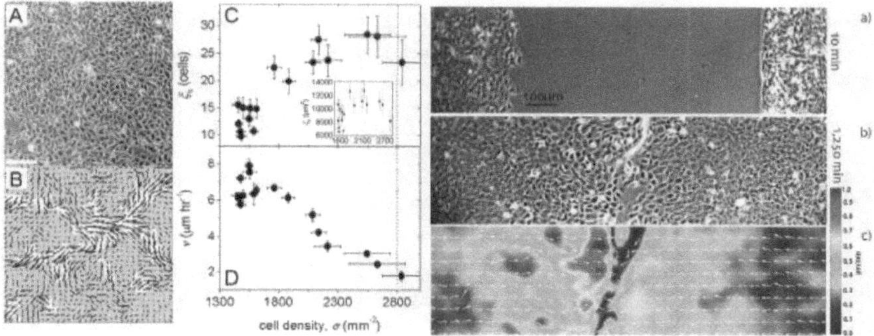

Figure 2.8: Cell jamming in 2D cell layers. Phase contrast images and velocity estimations via particle image velocity are shown. The left part of the figure is reprinted from [21] (Published by the National Academy of Sciences), where a slow down for increasing density in layers of epithelial-like MDCK cells was observed. The right part of the figure is reprinted from [22], where it was shown that two fronts epithelial-like MCF-10A do not mix. ©IOP Publishing Ltd and Deutsche Physikalische Gesellschaft. CC BY 3.0.

systems near a glass transition, and a dynamic structure factor reminiscent of glassy behaviour with decreasing self-diffusivity of short-wavelength motions and increasing cooperative long-wavelength fluctuations. They correlated this glassy slow-down with an increasing cell density in the layer. [21] Nnetu et al. reported in 2012, that fronts of MCF-10A cell layers in wound healing experiments do not mix after meeting, even though they are composed of the same cell type [22]. This indicates a solid-like behaviour of the cell layers, since fluids of the same materials are generally miscible. Later publications confirmed that the MCF-10A cells behave solid-like in densely-packed conditions [23, 94, 178].

With the existence of glass-like arrest being established, the search for the driving factors of the transition between the states of motility begun. I will discuss the theoretical approaches regarding this problem in the next chapter. One of the first proposed hypothesis with experimental evidence, was that maturing adhesion bonds between the cells cause friction, that slows the motion of the layer [27]. Garcia et al. measured the cellular motion in two-dimensional layers of immortalised human bronchial epithelial cells and found that the slow down in motion can not be rescaled on the cellular density of the system. They reported an ageing effect, that slowed-down the system more for older layers than explainable by the cell density alone. They correlated this ageing effect to an increasing fluorescence intensity of adhesion molecules in the layer and thus formulated the hypothesis of a friction-induced slow-down of the motion in tissues, caused by adhesion molecules. [27] I will discuss the effects of cell-cell adhesion further within this thesis, showing that a jamming transition is not necessarily correlated with increased adhesion. However, a decrease of cell-cell adhesion can unjam tissues by loss of coherence.

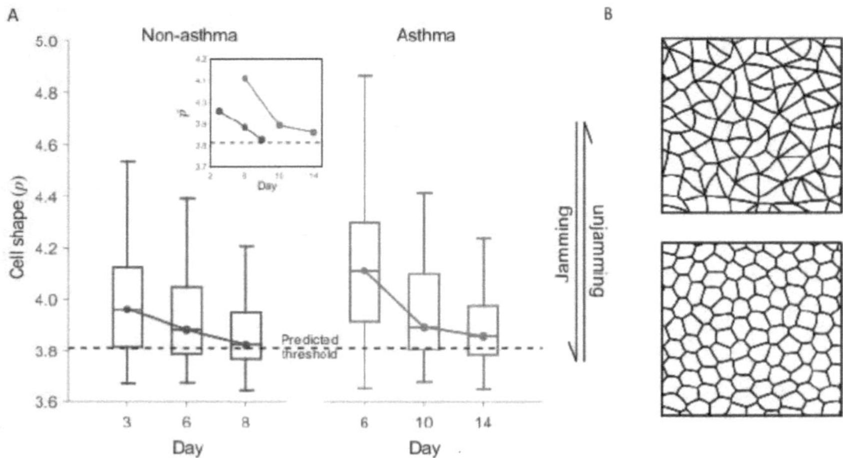

Figure 2.9: Development of airway epithelium compared between a healthy and an asthmatic condition. The healthy conditions have an arrest in cell motion, while the cells with asthmatic condition continue to move. The difference in the motility of the system is correlated with the cell shapes in the layer. Reprinted from [26]. ©2015 Springer Nature, license number 4998240029331.

The first publication that experimentally linked the cell shape in tissues with an arrest in motion was Park et al. in 2015 [26]. They studied primary human bronchial epithelial cells from asthmatic and non-asthmatic donors in a liquid/air interface culture. They observed a dynamic arrest for non-asthmatic airway epithelium, with glassy characteristics similar to those found by Angelini et al. [26, 21]. The motion of asthmatic airway epithelium required longer to slow down and never arrested completely [26]. All of the epithelial layers were confluent, at a volume fraction of one. Park et al. reported a correlation of the cell shapes in the epithelial layers with their state of motility, as previously predicted by vertex models [30, 26]. There have been further studies, that connected the cell jamming transition with the cell shapes of the tissue [179, 180, 181, 178, 182, 183]. It was found, that the shape distribution of tissues follows geometrical constrains, that have been first described for granular material [179, 184]. However, all of these studies were performed using two-dimensional epithelial sheets and studied the average cell shape and amount of motion. The work in this thesis expands the horizon, by showing that the cell shapes are also connected to jamming in three-dimensional tissue (see chapter 4.4) and by studying the rearrangement dynamics of individual cells depending on the properties of their neighbourhood, providing explicit insight to the underlying factors of the caging effect (see chapter 4.3).

The concept of cell jamming describes a system, where cells are caged by their neighbours, but can break out of these cages, given enough activity. This is a similar concept to a yield stress on a macroscopic level. It is therefore not surprising, that the system can fluidise if the activity of the cells gets increased. This has been done recently with RABA5, an endocytic protein, which enhances endosomal trafficking and macropinocytic internalization and thereby increasing traction and protrusions which are correlated with the cell velocity [185, 186, 187, 188]. The molecular and biological processes involved are complex and more than just an increase in activity can contribute to these findings, like a decrease in adhesion by increased turnover of adhesion bonds [185, 189]. Nevertheless, these findings are principally connected to cell activity and show a pathway for unjamming, that also might be connected to cancer [185, 189]. The connection between cell jamming and a decrease in traction and therefore presumably activity has also been made recently in the absence of RABA5 treatment [190].

In many cases, an unjamming of a previously jammed system has been connected to a correlated motion with very long correlation lengths, that has often been described as flocking [24, 191, 164, 185, 186, 94, 187, 188, 178]. The high cluster size in the dynamic behaviour indicates, that the systems are still close to the jamming transition, considering the analogy to colloidal glasses and jammed systems [192, 193]. This becomes appreciable by considering that cells within the large collectively moving clusters still have to move coordinated with their neighbours. In this sense, most of the cells within these systems are still caged and the system is close to the cell jamming transition, even though the velocities of motion could potentially be high. These considerations underline, that a jammed layer losing its boundary, for example in a wound healing experiment, will migrate collectively into open space, connecting cell jamming and collective motion [22, 24, 191, 94]. This line of thinking again motivates the analysis of individual cell rearrangements depending on the cellular environment as a direct source of the underlying factors of the caging effect in cell jamming (see chapter 4.3).

There have been drastically less studies of jammed cellular behaviour in three-dimensional tissue. Schötz et al, was the first publication that showed a glass-like behaviour of cellular motion in confluent three-dimensions explants from zebrafish embryos [25]. They showed that the mean squared displacement curves had a sub-diffusive exponent and that the so-called non-Gaussian parameter exhibited a peak typical for glassy behaviour [25]. Despite these microscopic indications of cell jamming, the macroscopic rheology was still consistent with fluid behaviour, showing an initial elastic response followed by viscous fluid-like behaviour in tissue surface tensiometer experiments and fluid-like spheroid fusions [25]. In another important publication in this regard, Mongera et al. showed cell jamming during the embryonic step of vertebrate body axis elongation [53]. They estimated the yield stress of the system and showed a dependency on N-cadherin adhesion and the volume fraction of the tissue [53]. The unjamming using RABA5 treatment was also checked for three-dimensional spheroids, but mostly described as a correlated rotation of the spheroid, which is consistent with the cells still being caged [188]. It is clear, that more research towards cell jamming in three-dimensional tissue is needed. It is shown, that cell jamming can have a macroscopic rheological effect in cell spheroids and that cell jamming correlates with the cell shape in three dimensions. It is shown that the nucleus shape has a strong correlation with the cell shape and motility, giving a physical underpinning to the measure of pleomorphism of cell nuclei used in cancer diagnosis.

2.2.3 Theories of cell jamming

There are different theoretical approaches modelling for cellular jamming. In this chapter I will summarise these theories and connect them to experimental findings in order to evaluate there claims. The earliest theory, that tried to explain cellular jamming did so in analogy to granular jamming [28]. They modelled cells as self-propelled soft particles and observed fluid-like behaviour for low volume fractions of cells and a jammed state for high volume fractions above $\Phi = 0.842$ [28]. This system can behave fluidly even for high volume fractions, when the activity of the particles is high enough, in analogy to overcoming a yield stress [28]. Below the volume fraction associated with jamming, there is a part of the phase diagram, where the system shows giant number fluctuations corresponding to collective movement, which were also observed in similar models studying collective motion [194, 195, 196, 197]. These types of models can be extended to include contact inhibition of locomotion, which changes quantitative results, but does not change the qualitative behaviour [198]. The deficiency of these models that are analogue to granular jamming is that they always predict a jammed behaviour or yield stress for confluent tissue, which exists at volume fraction one. As described in chapter 2.2.1, there are many tissues that behave fluidly without showing any signs of a yield stress. Since a focus of this thesis is the jamming transition within fully confluent tissue, these models are not best suited to describe this process. However, they could be useful to describe the behaviour of epithelial-like cells in situations with a lower volume fraction of cells.

There are models, that try to describe confluent tissue with extremely soft particles [27]. They require a large set of parameters like the strength of motility force f_0, a mean persistence time τ, the potentials of repulsion and attraction, a stiffness k, an equilibrium distance r_n and a background friction λ [27]. The disadvantage of using this many parameters is that many different conclusions could be drawn, depending on the position in the parameter space, which makes it difficult to evaluate the theory. The model by Garcia et al., that I highlighted here is interesting for this thesis, because it predicts a jamming transition for increased adhesion inducing friction between cells [27]. The publication presenting this model contains motivating experiments, in which an ageing effect in epithelial monolayers was observed and connected this with an increasing amount of adhesion bonds in fluorescence images [27]. A comparable system in this thesis has also shows an ageing effect, but I found no increase of adhesion connected to it, similar to other recent studies [190]. There are a multitude of other potential reasons for an ageing effect of the cell layer, as I discuss in more detail in the results section.

Vertex or Voronoi models are better suited to represent confluent tissue, than typical particle models. The tissue can be partitioned by a Voronoi tessellation around the cell centres or the connecting lines between vertices, which represent the outlines of cells in tissues. On can assign these cells an energy function. The one typically used Hamiltonian for a layer of N cells has been defined by Farhadifar et al. [199] and a simplified version has been used by Bi et al. to simulate jammed cell behaviour [30]:

$$E = \sum_{i=1}^{N} E_i = \sum_{i=1}^{N} K_{A,i} \left(A_i - A_{i,0}\right)^2 + K_{P,i} \left(P_i - P_{i,0}\right)^2 \tag{2.1}$$

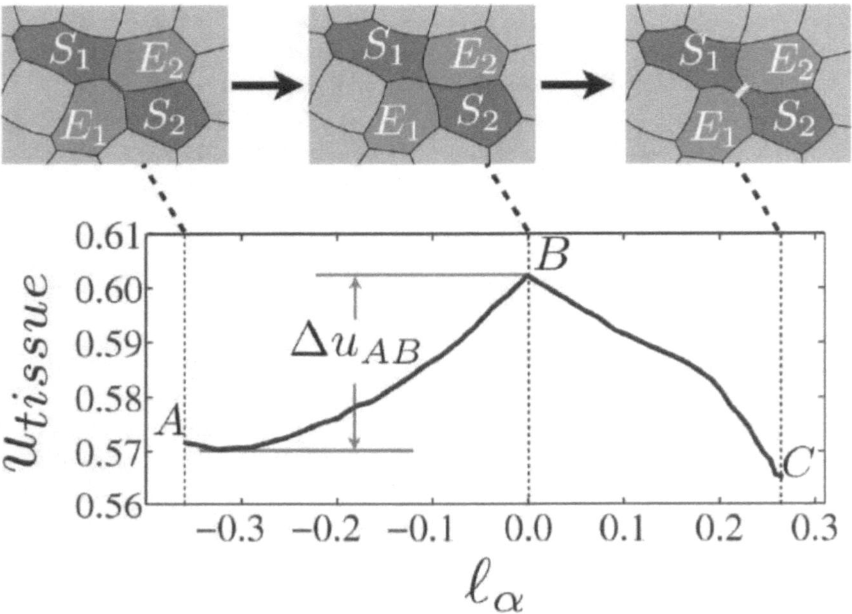

Figure 2.10: The upper row illustrates a T1 transition inside a confluent cell layer. The lower row shows change in the energy of the layer during this transition, depicting an energy barrier for this system. Thereby l_α describes the length of the edge changing during the T1-transition depicted above. Reprinted from [30] with permission from Royal Society of Chemistry (Order licence ID 1093936-1).

Here, A_i and P_i are the area and perimeter of each cell, while $A_{i,0}$ and $P_{i,0}$ are the intrinsically preferred area and perimeter of the respective cells. $K_{A,i}$ and $K_{P,i}$ are the area and perimeter moduli, respectively, and represent how strongly the cells prefer these areas and perimeters by exerting an energy penalty for deviations from those preferred values. The quadratic area term in the Hamiltonian represents a the incompressibility, resistance to being deformed perpendicular to the layer and an adhesion to the substrate. The quadratic term in the perimeter represents the interplay between cell-cell adhesion and cortical contractility, whereby a high amount of adhesion tends to elongate cells and a high amount of cortical contractility tends to round up the cells. [200] If one assumes a homogeneous cell layer ($A_0, P_{i,0}$ are constant), most of the parameters can be factored out and the only relevant parameter left, describing the system is the dimensionless preferred shape parameter $p_0 = P_0/\sqrt{A_0}$ [31]. Bi Dapeng and co-workers observed energy barriers for T1-transitions, which are the minimal topological transition required for cell rearrangement in simulated layers that had a preferred cell shape lower than the critical cell shape of $p^* \approx 3.81$ [30] (see figure 2.11). These energy barriers can be interpreted as the yield stress of a jammed system. This translates to a shape-dependent rigidity transition of the layer, when the preferred cell shape got round enough [31].

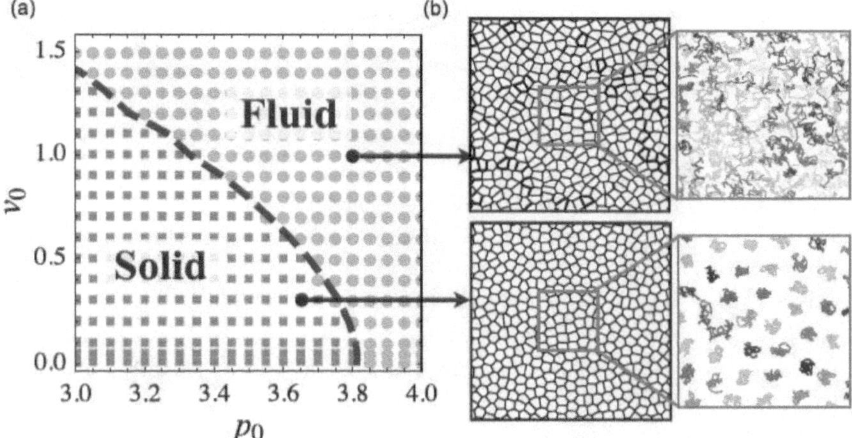

Figure 2.11: a) Phase diagram of simulations of the Voronoi model with self-propelled cells. Blue dots represent solid states and yellow dots represent fluid-like states with a blue dashed line representing the transition between these states. b) Example configurations of simulated cell layers with exemplary tracks. Reprinted from [32]. CC BY 3.0.

One can qualitatively explain these findings with changing degrees of freedom in the layer. If cells can be elongated, there are more possibilities to arrange cells, which they can use to rearrange themselves without requiring cells to occupy configurations that are energetically unfavourable. Reversely, if the whole neighbourhood of cells is round, there is almost no possibility to leave it without any of the cells to elongate, which would require energy representing a yield stress. This model became prominent, because of experimental results that linked cell jamming and the cell shape, as discussed in the previous chapter [26, 179, 180, 181, 178, 182, 183]. From a biological perspective, this model predicts a jamming of cells with high actin contractility and low cell adhesion. The tissue still has to stay confluent for the model to be able to describe it, which means that drastic decrease of adhesion can not be represented. A verification of this model by checking these biological predictions gets complicated by the fact that many prominent adhesion molecules interact with the actin cortex beneath and remodel it [63, 64, 65]. I will provide some context for the value of the shape parameter. The packing that has the lowest mean shape parameter of cells with $p = 3.72$ is the hexagonal packing, sometimes called honeycomb packing after the corresponding conjecture [201]. The mean shape parameter resulting from a Voronoi-tessellation of random seeds is $p \approx 4.22$.

Further studies of this model analysed the behaviour of this model with self-propelled Voronoi cells. Thereby, the velocity of the cells is governed by the following overdamped equation:

$$\frac{\mathrm{d}\vec{r_i}}{\mathrm{d}t} = -\mu \nabla_i E + v_0 \vec{n}_i \tag{2.2}$$

The mobility is denoted as μ, the self-propulsion velocity is called v_0 and $\vec{n}_i$ is the polarity vector along which the self-propulsion force is exerted. Unsurprisingly, it was reported that an activity of cells shifts the required preferred shape parameter for jamming to lower values [32]. The critical value of $p^* \approx 3.81$ is recovered for cell velocities near zero. A phase diagram displaying these effects is shown in figure 2.11. On the right side of this figure exemplary cell configurations and cell tracks are shown. The simulated cell tracks cross each other often in the fluid system, while the cells in the solid system stay mostly at their place, even if occasional rearrangements can occur.

Other interesting findings regarding this model include that disperse distributions of preferred parameter in the layer increase the critical shape parameter required for jamming, shifting the rigidity transition to higher values [202]. It has also been connected to collective motion and flocking, which is reflected in my discussion about this topic in the previous chapter [187]. Recently, cell jamming has been simulated for Voronoi tessellations in the three-dimensional case [46]. The Hamiltonian is the same, with the relevant cell parameters being the cell volume instead of the cell area and the cell surface instead of the cell perimeter. Consequently, the three-dimensional shape parameter is defined by $s = \frac{V}{S^{2/3}}$. It was not a priori clear, that the jammed behaviour of this model was transferable to three dimensions, because there cells have more degrees of freedom in higher dimensions. The observed jammed behaviour in the model requires the freezing of some of those degrees of freedom by residual stresses caused by cells being unable to achieve their preferred shape [46]. Merkel and Manning reported a critical shape parameter for three-dimensional Voronoi cells of $s_0 \approx 5.41$.

Cell jamming transitions can also be modelled in cellular Potts models which represent cells as regions in a lattice and stochastically evolve the system. The Hamiltonians used are qualitatively similar, describing interfacial tension caused by cortex tension and adhesion, as well as area incompressibility and active motility [203]. The results are qualitatively similar, reporting a jammed state for round cells and a fluid state for cells that prefer an elongated shape. The critical preferred cell shape marking this transition in two dimensions for Potts models is $p*_{Potts} = 4.9$ [203]. This is much higher than the critical value for Voronoi cells, which is not too surprising, as the Voronoi tessellation does not include fluctuations of the perimeter and minimises the observed cell shapes. In all of these models, the effect of cell density is unexplored, because they are build in a dimensionless fashion. There are results in this thesis, that indicate that the number density of cells in confluent tissue, influences the cell jamming transition.

Another interesting model, that has been published recently, models cells as deformable polygons [47]. While it has the disadvantage of containing many parameters, that allow potential fudging, it was able to reproduce the shape-dependent jamming transition in confluent layers and extend it to the case of volume fractions lower than one [47]. For absolutely round cells, the critical volume fraction is at $\frac{\Phi_J}{\Phi_{max}} \approx 0.81$ [47]. Even if it is potentially possible, the influence of the number density has not been studied in this model yet.

Chapter 3

Materials and Methods

I used several different biophysical methods to characterise cells and tissues during the jamming transition. The methods of cell culture, spheroid preparation and microscopy are standard in the field and can be reproduced by consulting the protocol section A. I employed spheroid fusion experiments in order to investigate the macroscopic rheological properties of densely packed three-dimensional tissues. The procedure of the spheroid fusion analysis can be comprehended by reading the publication of Flenner et al. [14]. Optical stretcher measurements were employed to investigate mechanical single cell properties of cells in different states of motility. These measurements are also state of the art and can be understood by consulting previous publications [72, 204, 205, 206] and the protocol section A.6. In the following part, I will concentrate on the methods that I have developed during the research for this thesis as well as the machine learning approach, which is adapted from the current literature, but contains intricacies that have to be explained more thoroughly.

3.0.1   Cell tracking

One of the main goals of this thesis was to study the effects of the local environment of cells in tissues on their state of motility, as well as the tissue dynamics during the transition from fluid-like cell behaviour to jammed tissue. This is not possible with particle image velocimetry (PIV), which is the prevalently used method to asses cell movement within tissues. It correlates the movement of features in the images series over time and thereby generates flow fields, that can give statistical information about the dynamics of the tissue. These statistical measures assume an unchanged behaviour over the time, they average and therefore are not well suited to describe the process of the transition and limit the temporal resolution. Furthermore, these flow fields can not be assigned to individual cells, limiting the spatial resolution drastically. Many of these problems can be solved by tracking of cells via their nucleus signal, as it allows to describe the motility of cells directly compared to their neighbours and even provides estimates of the structural properties of the environment.

In order to allow tracking, the cell nuclei were stained with vital $0.1\,\mu M$ SiR-DNA (Spirochrome) stain and imaged in a time series. The tracking procedure was varied depending on the properties of the imaged time series and the requirements on the quality of the resulting tracks. For the experiments of the dynamic with epithelial-like layers, presented in the chapters 4.1 and 4.3, the local cell rearrangements were the focus and the cell tracks were also used to estimate local structural properties, which both require the correct tracking of nearly all cells. These high requirements on the necessitated a custom identification of the nuclei, adapted to the specific image properties, prior to the tracking of the nuclei via TrackMate [207]. For the experiments presented in chapter 4.2 and the tumour pieces presented in chapter 4.4.3 only the dynamical state of the system was of interested and ensemble statements were sufficient. Therefore, it was not a requirement to track every cell inside the tissue and the built-in particle detection of TrackMate [207] turned out to be of sufficiently good quality. For the live imaging of spheroids presented in chapter 4.4.1, the image quality of the time series did not allow for a sufficient quality of automated tracking of nuclei and consequently a small subset of nuclei were tracked by hand.

Larger regions without nuclei (for example wounds in wound healing experiments) produce false positive cell positions in the procedure described below, because of the use of adaptive thresholds. Therefore, those are excluded by a mask found by high values of an entropy map of the phase contrast image of the cell layer. These high entropy regions are liberally dilated and small holes are filled.

The thresholding of the nuclei signal is done by multiple filters which all allow too many pixels individually, but give a good representation when combined. Please note, that histogram based thresholding for example with an Otsu criteria, do not work well, because the intensity of the fluorescence value can be quite different for different cells, especially for different cell lines or in different z-slices of 3D-experiments. The first two filters used are two median based adaptive threshold filters with different window sizes. One window size is roughly a nucleus radius and the second one is 25x larger. Additionally a mean based adaptive threshold with a window size of roughly a nucleus diameter is used. A good way to separate nearby nuclei is to sort out pixel with a high entropy value. This discards all border pixels of the nuclei.

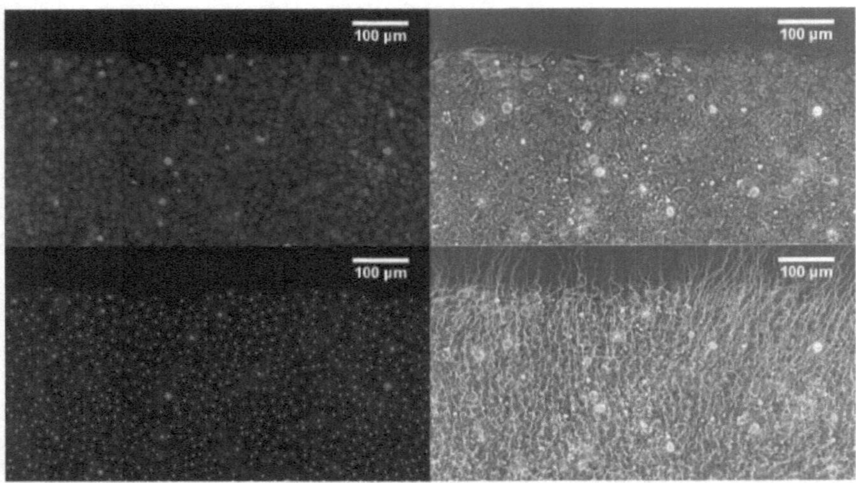

Figure 3.1: Part of a wound healing experiment of MCF-10A cells, depicted directly after removal of the wound healing insert. The experiment has high demands on the automated image processing, since the layer is very dense and the nucleus signal is slightly blurred. Upper Left: The signal of the stained nuclei (SiR-DNA). Upper Right: Overlay of phase contrast and nuclei signal. Lower Left: Grey Scale of nuclei signal overlaid with the detected nuclei centres. Lower Right: The original image overlaid with 6h tracks of the cell movement.

This procedure produces already a good black and white representation of the nuclei signal. It is finalised by morphological opening and deleting structures too small to be nuclei, followed by the closing of small holes inside the features, which can occur due to the adaptive threshold with a small window size. The middle of the nuclei is found as maxima of Gaussian-smoothed distance distribution to the outside of the structures. This procedure does separate two neighbouring nuclei, which are attached by a small bottleneck.

The nuclei centres are than tracked with the FijI plugin TrackMate [207, 208, 209].

MCF-10A cells, which build up the epithelial-like layers for the experiments that required a previous nuclei detection, usually move quite slowly in a closed layer. A maximum step size of 12 μm for tracks with image sequences with an image every 10 minutes works well. A maximum gap of two frames is allowed to give some leeway if a nuclei is not detected in one frame. On the other hand, only tracks spanning at least 20 frames are kept to sort out misdetections, because those are usually quite short. This sorts out some of the correctly tracked cells, whose tracks are interrupted, because nuclei were not found for a few frames, but this happens rarely and it is still better to exclude some correctly tracked nuclei than to include false tracks. The quality of the tracking is checked by eye for each experiment.

As already mentioned, the open source FijI plugin TrackMate is able to detect the nuclei by itself, if the image quality is good enough and it is not required that absolutely every nucleus is detected and tracked [207, 208, 209]. This approach is used for the data presented in chapter 4.2 and chapter 4.4.3. It is best to try different parameters during the tracking process and check the results by eye in order to minimise the tracking errors for each data set. A good starting point for the spot size of nuclei is a diameter of 10 µm, which was used for the experiments in both of those chapters. After the initial detection, TrackMate allows the user to generate filters to remove misdetected spots. This a very useful step to improve the quality of the tracks and I would advise anyone doing it to invest time and try different filter combinations. It is best to look at the detections that potential filters would sort out to asses their usefulness.

The advantage of using the particle detection of the tracking software is that one can use the features of the detected spots to improve the linkage of the spots between the different images of the time series. I employed a penalty for differences in the estimated spot diameter, the median spot intensity and the standard deviation of the spot intensity in the linking process to reduce rare occasions, where tracks jumps from one nucleus to another even further. This allows also to increase the maximum linkage distance to a value slightly larger than the maximal frame-to-frame velocities. If one adjusts it too large the occasions where tracks jump from cell to cell, instead of disappearing when a detection goes wrong, increases and will be visible by eye. It is useful to allow short gaps in the tracks to accommodate some instances where the nuclei are not detected in a few frames. The longest allowed gaps for my tracking process was 2 frames. Inspecting the tracks, it becomes apparent that most of the misdetections are present in very short tracks, because the wrong tracks do not follow real cells nuclei and therefore disappear fast. This means that it is useful to sort out short tracks in order to increase the quality of the remaining ones. I sorted out at least all of the tracks that are shorter than 10 frames.

TrackMate allows for the export of tracks as a structure in a .xml file. This can be loaded in any program allowing data analysis, which was in my case Matlab. The .xml file that TrackMate produces contains a structure with all approved tracks and for each track a list of the frames and positions. It is useful to implement additional structures like a list of each frame containing the tracks that are present in them and lists of the neighbours of each track at each time point. The neighbours of cells can be detected as the tracks that share two vertices in the Voronoi-tessellation of all track positions in one frame. These Voronoi-tessellations can also be used to estimate structural properties of confluent epithelial layers like the cell number density and cell shape [210]. Since the tessellation in this case is done around nucleus centres and not the central point of the cell, the resulting cell shapes tend to err on the side of more elongated shapes compared to the usual model of Voronoi-tessellations. It is still a useful approach to dynamically estimate the structure of the tissue, as will become clear in the result section.

There are several potential pitfalls for an otherwise conceptually easy analysis. One should limit the data set to a region with enough distance to the edge of the image and if one uses a Voronoi-tessellation, only those cells whose corner vertices are all inside the original image should be used. In three-dimensional data the z-resolution is usually worse than the x/y-resolution and it is worth to check if the noise of a measure reduces drastically, if one only uses the projection of the movement. Since it is known that cell proliferation and death can fluidise a system [211, 212], one can consider to only use tracks where no neighbours appear or disappear in the time period for the dynamical analysis. This is the 'ground state' of the motility state.

3.0.2   Cell segmentation

The core question of this thesis is what features of the tissue cause its dynamic behaviour. At least from a coarse-grained perspective, the structure of the tissue is the prime candidate [163, 32, 47, 213]. The structure of static images of tissues that have known differences in their state of motility is thereby of great interest. In this section, I will describe the process of segmenting cell shapes from images containing the relevant structural information. I will focus on the approach in 3D tissue used for analysis presented in chapter 4.4.2. The approach in 2D, used in chapter 4.2.1, follows the same qualitative algorithm, except for the error control.

It is necessary to estimate the structure of the local environment by a Voronoi-tessellation during time series of moving cells, mainly because of the added photo-toxicity of too many simultaneous fluorescence images over a long time period.

The segmentation image analysis was done using a self-written MatLab algorithm whose steps are described in the following: The starting point of this segmentation algorithm are 3D fluorescence images (stacks) of cell aggregates. I stained the nuclei with the DNA stain SiR-DNA. As information about the cell outlines, I used actin staining. Actin assembles beneath the cell membrane to a cortex, which gives boundary information. The nuclei stain serves as a proxy for "cell center" information.

I used nuclei information as a starting point. From this, a gradient map of the actin signal was computed and used as input to a watershed algorithm – which is run from the "wells" that I obtained by the cell center signal. The cells have to be optically cleared and the signal quality has to be good (low noise, achieved by high-NA imaging). A small distance between the z-stacks is also necessary to the segmentation to deliver satisfactory results. The slightly declining fluorescence intensity level in upper parts of the spheroids was corrected by subtracting a morphologically opened image, and then re-adjusting the intensity afterwards. An adaptive median filter lowers salt-and-pepper-noise. The intensity of dark z-slices was increased to match the mean intensity of brighter z-slices.

Next, the empty background is detected to find the boundary of the spheroid. I used an entropy filter alongside with the actin signal, which was followed by a Gaussian window filter. The filter kernel was chosen larger than a cell size to ensure that the spheroid is detected, but no noise or single cell structures. The spheroid as such is detected by simple thresholding and image filling.

One of the most decisive steps is a good nuclei detection. If multiple nuclei are mis-registered as a single one the cell segments will be combined to form one larger segment, defying the purpose of the whole segmentation routine.

The nuclei detection works similar to the one described in the cell tracking chapter. The nuclei are found by adaptive thresholding: In order to minimise false positives, the detected foreground has to be above the threshold of multiple window sizes. The foreground is smoothed by the morphological processes of dilation and erosion. Small holes in the nuclei mask are filled. Connected regions that are too small to be cell

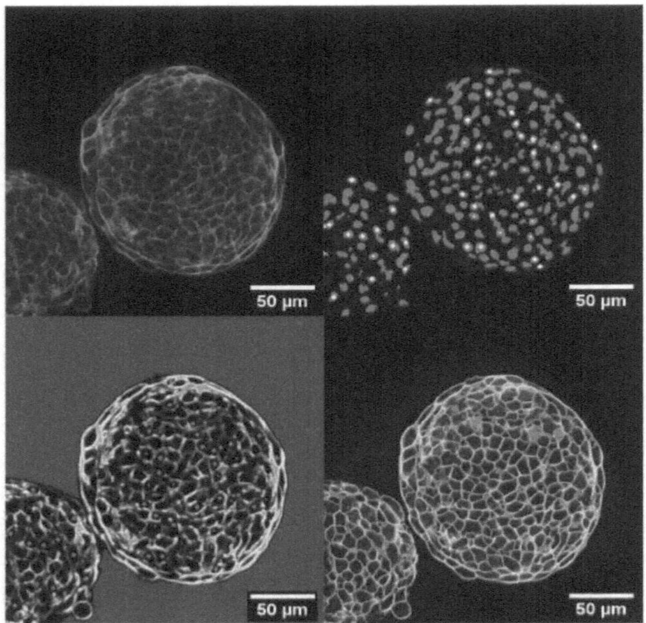

Figure 3.2: The segmentation routine. Upper Left: Original fluorescence data. Actin, green, and nuclei, blue. Upper Right: Nuclei detection. Nuclei are blue. Detected nuclei are red. Segmentation seeds, white. Not all seeds are visible, as most of them lie in planes slight above or below this exemplary slice. Lower left: The water shedding is based on actin and nucleus signals, and on gradients of the actin signal. Blue, spheroid-free background. Red, nuclei seeds. Lower right: The post-processed actin and nuclei signals (green and blue) overlayed with the outlines as found by the segmentation routine (red).

nuclei are ignored.

One problem is that nuclei that are too close together are sometimes not properly separated. Together, they often form ellipsoids connected by a neck. To separate them, I used a small helping algorithm: The distance map of the detected foreground pixels to the background was calculated. This map was then smoothed and its maxima were found. This routine was inspired by[214].

These maxima serve as seeds for the cell segmentation. They were dilated, with spheres much smaller than the typical nuclei radius to help fuse seeds which were very close to each other. This ensured that seeds of different nuclei almost never fused, leading to seed maps of the nuclei that I intensively checked for credibility.

The seeds mark the positions of, or rather the inside, of cells, but not the boundaries between the cells. The next step uses a gradient map of the actin signal. This gradient map was smoothed with a Gaussian filter (this time using a smaller window size) to avoid ending up with two different maxima lines per actin cortex. Afterwards, the actin signal was added to the gradient map as additional border information and half of the value of the nucleus signal was removed, because the nuclei indicate center positions. This map was superimposed with negative infinity on the location of the nuclei seeds and the previously detected cell-free background and used as the basis for water shedding.

The watershed lines yield a connected network of cell boundaries. I then filtered out some misdetections by (1), their small size – much smaller than a typical cell size – or by (2) being devoid of any seed (i.e. in the case of a small "enclosure" with no nucleus in it). Misdetections were added to outline volumes, which were later shrinked again.

Another step to ensure the quality of the whole segmentation was to check which seeds lead to misdetections, to discard them in the first place and re-run the whole routine with a "corrected" set of seeds.

It is a challenging to estimate the errors of the segmentation, because it is not practical to correct a three-dimensional cell segmentation by hand. In order to produce a test for the segmentation with known cell shapes, artificial spheroids were produced. These propose similar challenges to spheroids analysed in chapter 4.4.2. The artificially generated nuclei have different sizes and are close to each other, sometimes even overlapping. This overlap does not occur in reality, but the resolution limit of the confocal microscope frequently leads to apparently overlapping nuclei. The noise added to the synthetic data appears larger than the noise in the confluent slides. The synthetic data and its segmentation, which was not adjusted from the algorithm used for the real spheroid stacks, are visualised by a slice though the equatorial plane on the left side of figure 3.3. The segmentation appears to correctly line up with the cell boundaries most of the time, although some errors are visible.

The right side of figure 3.3 depicts an evaluation of the data quality with comparison

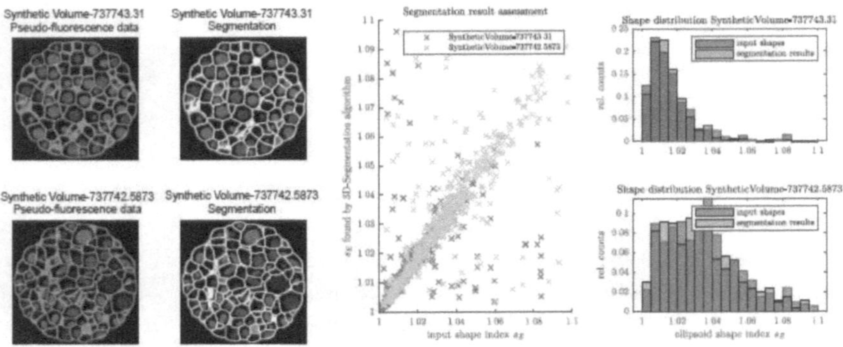

Figure 3.3: Test of cell segmentation on synthetic data. The left images show equatorial plains of synthetic three-dimensional data with round cell shapes on top and more elongated cell shapes on the bottom. The nucleus representation is coloured red, the actin representation green and the outlines of segmented cells are white. The graph in the middle depicts the one-to-one dependency of the segmented cell shape on the known synthetic cell shapes. Histograms of the known synthetic shape indices and the estimation using segmented cells are on the right side.

of the measured and known cell shape of each cell in the middle and histograms of both distributions on the right side. The measure representing the cell shape is the three dimensional cell shape index of the ellipsoid with the same second moments as the cell shape, normed to one for spheres $s_E = (36\pi)^{-1/3} \cdot S_E \cdot V_E^{-2/3}$. This measure is used to minimise artefacts from misdetection of the surface and arbitrariness from the exact calibration of the segmentation code. Most of the cells of the synthetic volume were segmented well and have the same, or nearly the same, cell shape index s_E as the known segments, visualised by a strongly populated region along the identity line in the comparison graph of figure 3.3. There are misdetections present displayed by the cells that fall away from the line, but those are comparably few in number. Since the goal is to identify ensemble differences and not the exact shape index of each cell for individual comparisons, the histograms entail the main message. The distributions of cell shapes are replicated quite reliably and the algorithm is clearly robust enough to distinguish the differences of the cell shape distribution between these spheroids.

Figure 3.4 depicts an estimation of the influence of noise in the original data on the segmented cell shapes, characterised by their cell shape index. The forms of noise

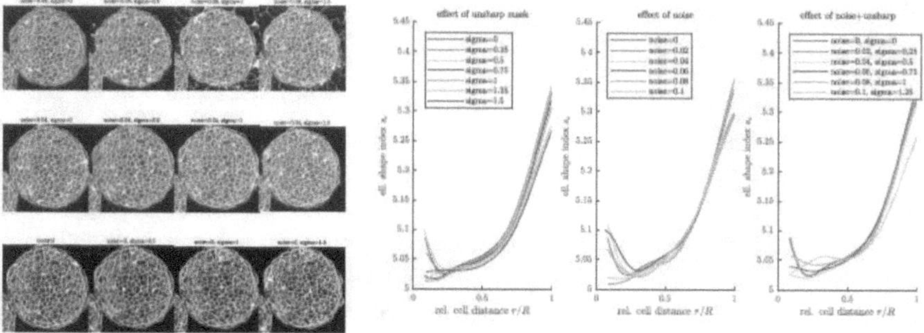

Figure 3.4: Three-dimensional cell segmentation with added Gaussian smoothing and white noise. The left images contain equatorial plains of an exemplary MCF-10A spheroid with increasing amount of Gaussian smoothing, representing worse image resolution, to the right and increasing amount of white noise, representing worse fluorescence quality, in upwards direction. On the right side, average cell shapes indices in dependence on the distance of the cell to the center are plotted for the different amounts of noise.

present in the original data are the limit of optical resolution and the microscopy process, which is a convolution with the point spread function and has a roughly similar effect to the additional smoothing with a Gaussian kernel [215]. The other kind of noise in the image is the white noise in the camera compared to the fluorescence signal. This can be increased by adding random (white) noise. It is visible, that the cell segmentation gets worse for increasing levels of noise, but retains its core characteristics quite long even for extraordinary amounts of noise. The regions that seem to suffer most are the regions on the edge of the spheroid.

For different amounts of each kind of noise, the right side of figure 3.4 shows distributions of cell shape indices that were averaged with a Gaussian kernel depending on the relative distance to the center of the spheroids. One peculiar effect for this specific spheroid is the small increase of the cell shape for cells very near the center of the spheroid. This is presumably caused by the low statistic of a spherical shell with very small radius and random chance, but interestingly it persists for many of the levels of added noise, indicating that the segmentation is quite robust in the regime. The overall behaviour of the cell shape index, meaning the core/shell structure, is never changed with the added noise levels even when they reach extremely high values, proving that the segmentation is robust enough to capture the structural features of the analysed spheroids.

The error estimation is much easier in two dimensions. In order to test the algorithm used in chapter 4.2.1, the wrongfully detected shapes of exemplary images were corrected by hand and the resulting shape distributions were compared. The automatic segmentation reflects the reality quite well. The differences between the corrected versions is typically much smaller than the sample variations. The largest difference between the mean cell shape index of an automated segmentation and the manual corrected version was $\Delta p = 0.07$, while the standard variation of the cell shape indices in this ensemble was $\sigma(p) = 0.76$. The estimated cell sizes barely differed. The errors in the cell shape of the automatic segmentation let the sample appear more average – elongated cells appear rounder and round cells appear more elongated. The Nematic Order Parameter is slightly underestimated, because of the errors in the automatic segmentation. Again, these are only minor effects.

3.0.3 Machine learning

In the chapter analysing the rearrangement dynamics in epithelial-like monolayers, one of the fundamental questions is whether the structural properties of the layer regions dictate their ability to rearrange and which of these structural properties influence the dynamical behaviour the most. One of the tools used to tackle this question were machine learning algorithms, inspired by a similar approach for glasses [216, 217].

The kind of machine learning algorithm employed here are Random Forests algorithms, since they can robustly handle outliers and the problem of collinearity in input parameters [218]. The Random Forests algorithm consists of an adjustable number of decision trees that act as an statistical ensemble [218]. Each tree in a Random Forest is constructed based on a randomly chosen subsample of the input data. In each individual tree a prediction is made by splitting the data points so that the difference between the resulting groups is maximised. The overall prediction is then made by taking the prediction with the most votes. This procedure is called bagging [219].

This makes the Random Forests algorithm a robust and accurate classifier, hence a significant number of predictive models, represented by lowly correlated trees, provides generally better performance than individual models. During bagging, furthermore, a subset of randomly selected features is selected to grow the tree at each node of RF. In parallel to training, the algorithm measures the prediction performance by using cross-validation on what is called out-of-bag samples. Concretely, each tree is constructed by drawing a particular bootstrap sample. Whereas several training examples will be repeated in the sample, a certain number of training data will be excluded of the sample considering that bootstrapping is sampling with replacement. The excluded data compose then the out-of-bag sample. On average, Random Forest algorithms construct each tree utilizing roughly $1-e^{-1} \cong 2/3$ of the training data and abandoning $e^{-1} \cong 1/3$ as out-of-bag samples. The prediction performance can be validated from out-of-bag samples, hence they have not been involved in the construction of trees [220]. The Random Forest algorithm was implemented in Python by the RandomForestClassifier in the Scikit-learn library [221].

The input training set consisted of 500,000 data points of cells at one time point with known environment and known future dynamic. The test set contained 125,000 of such data points. Each cell was characterised by 46 structural parameters whose composition and relative importance is discussed in chapter 4.3.3. Moreover, 11 informational parameters were recorded for each cell. These parameters describe environmental stability and dynamics of the cell and were not used to train the algorithm. These informational parameters contain for example, the parameters *time confluent* and *time layer-like*, which were used to select confluent cells and cells in epithelial-like layers, respectively. To sort out cells that undergo cell division during observation I examined if a cell appears or disappears in neighbourhood within 2 hours. To construct a supervised task, the 20% fastest cells were determined based on different dynamic measures, but mostly on the values of D^2_{min} with $Rc = 100 \ \mu m \ dt = 2h$. Each cell within the 20% fastest rearranging cells was labelled with 1, the rest was labelled with 0. The training as well as the test set consisted of equal sized groups. As demonstrated in Table 3.1, the labelling of the cell dynamic using D^2_{min} with $Rc = 100 \ \mu m \ dt = 2h$ provides the highest accuracy.

The tunable parameters were optimised through 5-fold cross-validation to ensure generalisability [223]. As can be seen in Figure 3.5, the optimisation showed that 500,000 cells were enough to train the Random Forest algorithm to generalise well. Thereby, the minimum number of samples required to be at a leaf node, the minimum number of samples required to split an internal node, the number of features to consider when looking for the best split, and the maximum depth of the tree were set to 4, 2, 0.5, and 7, respectively. For the model in this study, the random state was set to 999. Initially, the algorithm was trained on the data set containing 46 structural parameters and

Parameter	Training accuracy	Test accuracy
D^2_{min} Rc=100 μm dt=2h [222]	75%	75%
p_{hop} [217]	74%	74%
D^2_{min} Rc=50 μm dt=1h [222]	69%	69%
number of new neighbors from far away	68%	67%
number of T1's in next hour	59%	59%
D^2_{min} Rc=100 μm dt=2h - time normalised	58%	57%
D^2_{min} Rc=100 μm dt=2h - time normalised to Gauss	57%	56%
hour of experiment	X	X
time confluent	X	X
time layer-like	X	X
no cells appear or disappear in nn within 2h	X	X

Table 3.1: Parameters used either for labeling (accuracy is given) or for selection of jammed cells and cells that do not undergo cell division during observation.

the experiment time. Subsequently, collinear parameters were deleted if their Pearson correlation coefficient was above 0.9, this procedure is called feature selection [224]. After feature selection we trained RF on 15 parameters that can be seen in Table 3.2 and whose classification accuracy as a function of training set size is shown in Figure 3.5.

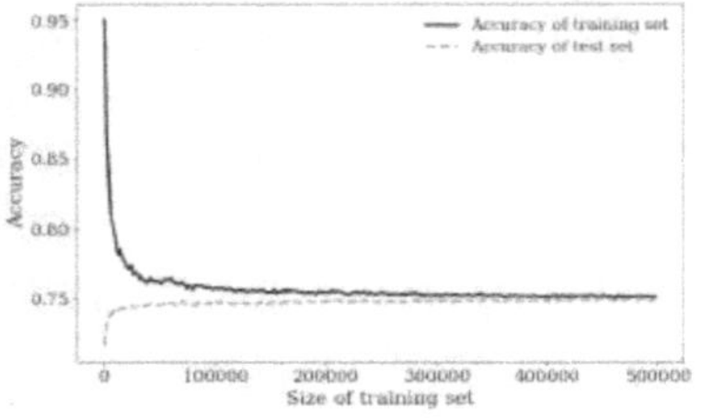
(a) Trained without *hour of experiment*.

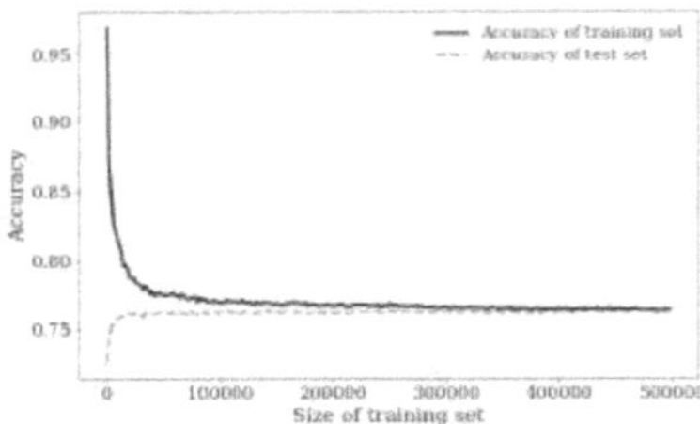
(b) Trained with *hour of experiment*.

Figure 3.5: Classification accuracy on the training and the test set as a function of training set size.

The classifiers were optimised in terms of accuracy, using permutation importance to estimate the importance of each parameter [225]. Permutation importance is a measure of the contribution of each parameter to the prediction accuracy that is computed during training. Hereby, the data of each parameter is permuted in the course of training

mean area of cell and direct neighbours
aspect ratio
change in area compared to 30 min before
change in shape parameter compared to 30 min before
mean shape within 200 μm
mean distance to 20th nn within 50 μm
std distance to 20th nn within 100 μm
std distance to 20th nn within 200 μm
mean density in cells per mm ^{2} within 100 μm
mean density in cells per mm ^{2} layer
mean shape layer
standart deviation of distance to 20th neighbour normed with mean
mean area of cell and direct neighbours - normed to frame
mean density in cells per mm ^{2} within 200 μm - normed to frame
hour of experiment - time of confluence

Table 3.2: Remaining parameters after performing feature selection.

of the Random Forest classifier for each tree. Permuting the data of each parameter simulates replacing it with random noise so that relevant features give significant effect on the prediction accuracy while irrelevant parameters have a minor impact on it. For each parameter, we calculate the accuracy on the out-of-bag sample of the cells without and with permutation. I do not use the out-of-bag error, which is commonly used to estimate the accuracy of the Random Forest classifier, since it tends to overestimate the true prediction error [226]. The according difference is recorded, averaged over all trees, and normalised by the standard error. This difference is then called the mean decrease in accuracy. These feature importances are the main result of this approach and discussed in chapter 4.3.3.

Chapter 4

Results

4.1 Signatures of cell jamming

This chapter provides a description of fundamental properties and processes during the cell jamming transition. These are interesting in their own right, but also necessary to understand the intricacies that are discussed in the later chapters. The cell jamming transition is discussed on the example of epithelial monolayers, which get denser over time, because of cell proliferation. Thereby, the cell layer transition from a fluid behaviour, allowing free rearrangement of cells within it, to a solid-like layer, where the cells are bound by their neighbours. Later chapters will not solely discuss the same system, but the concepts that are introduced here can be transferred and any differences will be clarified when they arise.

4.1.1 Dynamic arrest in epithelial cell layers

For the experiments described in this chapter, MCF-10A cells, whose nuclei were stained with SiR-DNA, were seeded on tissue culture treated polymer cover slips and observed over 3 days using a confocal laser scanning microscope with a 10 min interval between frames. The experiment was conducted in growth medium allowing the layer to get denser over time in order to study the dynamic arrest of the cell layer that occurs under these conditions.

Figure 4.1 gives an illustration of the cell behaviour during the experiment. It shows example sections of a layer in the sparse state(left) and in the densely packed state(right). Phase contrast images (gray), overlaid with the fluorescence signal of the nuclei in red and yellow indication lines of the tracks of nuclei movement within ±1.5 h. The nucleus movement is used as an approximation of the cell movement for these experiments. The tracking procedure is described in chapter 3.0.1.

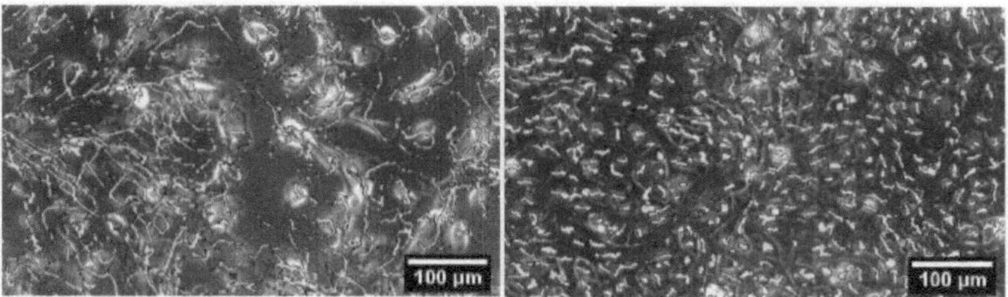

Figure 4.1: Images of epithelial-like MCF-10A cell layers. Phase contrast images are overlaid with the nucleus signal in red and yellow lines indicating the tracks of the cell nuclei within ±1.5 h. The left image shows a layer at the beginning of the experiment in a sparse and fluid state. The right image shows the same layer later in a dense and nearly arrested state.

In the sparse state on the left side, free space in-between the cells and lamellipodia are visible in the phase contrast image. The movement of the cells is barely restricted by their neighbours since there are many degrees of freedom due to the open space. Even if a cell is enclosed by other cells, those neighbours seldom are enclosed themselves and the force of a pushing cell can not be transferred through a tissue. The long tracks signify a comparably high cell velocity and the crossing of the tracks illustrate the possibility of cell rearrangements.

The phase contrast image in the right part of figure 4.1 shows no free spaces and relatively straight cell boundaries instead of the lamellipodia. The velocity of the cells is slowed down compared to the sparse state of the layer, illustrated by the shorter tracks. The tracks also do not cross each other and nearby tracks tend to be parallel, especially if they are long compared to the others. This indicates that a considerably large part of the motion is collective and not individual.

The nuclei positions, that were detected for the tracking algorithm can also be used for an estimation of cell features such as the cell size and the cell shape via a Voronoi-tessellation. In very sparse layers, such as the one shown on the left side of figure

4.1, the Voronoi-tessellation is very error prone especially for the cell shape, since it extends into the cell free territory. On the other hand, a Voronoi-tessellation provides a suitable approximation of cell shapes in confluent epithelial-like cell layers [210]. For this reason, most of following analysis, except the overall time evolution graphs include only data point from confluent layers. In any case, the confluent part of the data is the more important part for the shape estimation, because this is the region where theories predict a shape-dependent jamming transition at a volume fraction of 1 [30, 31, 32, 46].

The cell shape can be quantified by the shape index $p = P/\sqrt{A}$, a dimensionless parameter defined as the ratio of the perimeter P and the square root of the Area A. Consider the following examples as a guidance, what these two-dimensional shape parameter mean. A hexagonal packing produces shape indices of 3.72, the critical shape parameter for cell jamming in Vertex models is 3.81 and the mean shape parameter resulting from a Voronoi-tessellation of random seeds is 4.22.

It is intuitively clear, that sparse epithelial cells can rearrange freely, because the open space does not constrain the cells and allows for many degrees of freedom in the cell movement. The errors that are induced in the estimation of the cell shape by the tessellation around the nuclei tend to increase the shape index of the detected cells, since nuclei are not always in the middle of the cells and the added noise tends to shift the shape index towards those of a random configuration, which is significantly higher than the ordered structure of a confluent layer.

The left side of figure 4.2 depicts a Voronoi-tessellation of a typical, freshly confluent, layer of MCF-10A cells as a net of white lines. The red background shows the fluorescence signal from the SiR-DNA stain of the cell nuclei and the yellow lines indicate the nuclei movement within $\pm 1.5\,\mathrm{h}$. Shortly after the layer gets confluent, there is still a large variance in local cell number density visible in the layer, that partially overlaps with regions of round cell shapes. Of course, these statements are just anecdotal in this image, but they will be validated in the further analysis.

The mean shape parameter of cells within these epithelial-like layers decreases over time, while the cell number density increases. This is pictured in the right side of figure 4.2, where each line depicts one experimental scene. The mean cell shape parameter of the layer starts at a value of around 4.3 for early experiment times and low densities and steadily decreases to a value of roughly 4.0. The three different colours indicate three independent experiments on different days. The decrease in mean cell shape for increasing cell layer densities follows the same smooth curve for all experiments, but

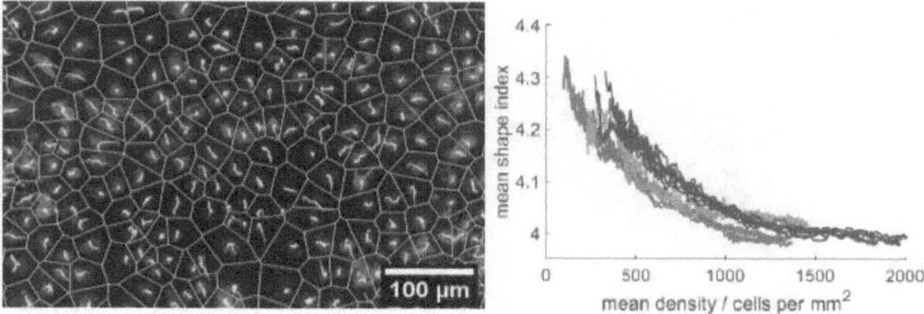

Figure 4.2: The left image shows the fluorescence of the stained nuclei of a section of an epithelial-like MCF-10A layer in red. The white lines build the Voronoi-tessellation around the detected nuclei centres of the current frame. The yellow lines depict the detracted tracks of the nuclei within $\pm 1.5\,\mathrm{h}$. The right image shows the time evolution of the mean cell number density and cell shape during the monolayer experiments estimated via the Voronoi-tessellation. The different colours indicate three independent experiments with seven independent scenes each.

is slightly shifted for experiments on different days, indicating the existence of further important parameters, that were not controlled in the experiment. These 21 scenes with a respective area of $2.5\,\mathrm{mm}^2$ contain 343660 detected tracks with about 35 million data points of nuclei positions within the tracks and are the basis of further analysis shown here and in chapter 4.3.

I will start with the basic description of the data set to enable a comprehensive understanding of the later presented analysis. Figure 4.3 depicts histograms of the properties of the local environments of the confluent time periods of the analysed MCF-10A layers, which will later be connected to the dynamical properties of the environments. It is visible in the left part of the figure, that the decrease in the mean cell shape, which was observed in figure 4.2, is mainly caused by the vanishing of highly elongated cells. The peak of histograms of local shape indices with the same local cell number density stays roughly similar. The shape parameter of the local environment appears stable, even in the logarithmic scale of the right plot in figure 4.2. Most of the data points have a change of lower than 0.05 within half an hour. The distribution is not radial symmetric. Most of the data points that have a strong change in the local shape parameter compared to half an hour ago have a similar reverse change within the next 30 min. This signifies that many of these strong changes are fluctuations and not snapshots of

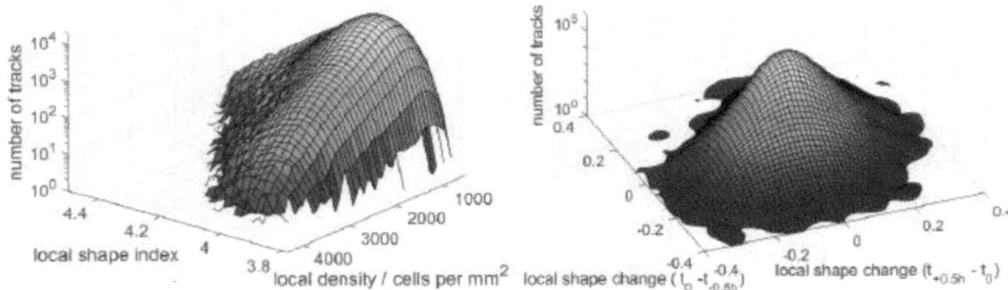

Figure 4.3: Histograms of the properties of local environments in the confluent part of the experiments. The left figure shows the histogram for the local cell number density and cell shape and the right figure illustrates the frequency of changes in the local cell shape within half an hour. The z-axes, showing the number of tracks is logarithmic. The histograms are smoothed with a Gaussian kernel.

a strong driven change within the local environment of the layer.

An illustration of the difference in kind of motion within confluent layers of MCF-10A cells is given by figure 4.4. At early experiment times and low densities, cells are able to move past each other and rearrange the cell layer. This is the upper time series in figure 4.4 and labelled as fluid region. In contrast, at later times and higher cells densities, the cell movement slows down visibly and cells are seldom able to move past their neighbours. The tracks of ± 1.5 hours in the lower time series show only small wiggling motion of the nuclei, within the cells, that are constrained by each other. When comparing the exemplary structures of the two time series, both the higher cell number density and order of the arrested region are appreciable. Note that the nuclei themselves have a rounder shape in the arrested region.

In order to quantify the rearrangements within the layer, one has to use a measure that incorporates the relative motion of cells. There is a discussion of multiple measures of the tissue dynamics in chapter 4.1.2. Here, I introduce the measure that turns out to be the most useful one at quantifying the dynamics of cell rearrangements, in order to be able to describe the overall time evolution of the tissue dynamics in the system. This measure is the magnitude of nonaffine displacement D_{min}^2, already commonly used in the analysis of glasses [222, 216, 217]. In contrast to MSD, it is not inherently a statistical measure, and can therefore make statements for individual cells, regions and

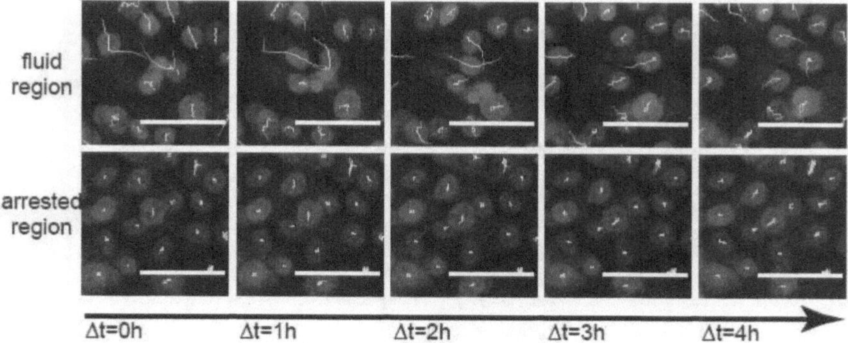

Figure 4.4: Example time series of cells in motile and arrested regions of the layer at differing starting times. The red background are fluorescence images of cell nuclei stained by SiR-DNA. The cell movement is indicated by yellow lines, corresponding to the tracks of the motion within $\pm 1.5\,$h. Scale bars represent $50\,\mu$m.

frames. It is therefore better able to resolve the transition between the dynamic states. The magnitude of nonaffine displacement D^2_{min}, used to characterise the rearrangement dynamics within the layer, is defined as:

$$D^2_{min}(i,t) = \min_{\Lambda}\{\frac{1}{z}\sum_{j}[R_{ij}(t+\Delta t) - \Lambda R_{ij}(t)]^2\} \tag{4.1}$$

This measure registers the movement of the cell i within the time frame Δt compared to the z close-by cells j and minimizes this over the tensor of all possible affine transformations Λ, thereby describing the relative rearrangement of the cell i at time t within the layer. $R_{ij}(\tau)$ is the distance between the cells i and j at time τ. I usually use $\Delta t = 2h$ and all cells j that are in a radius of 100 μm of cell i.

The time evolution of the cell rearrengment dynamics is shown in figure 4.5. The mean nonaffine displacement of each cell in the layer within 2 hours after each frame is plotted over the experiment time. Identical to figure 4.2, the 21 lines represent independent sections of MCF-10A layers and the three colours represent three different experiment dates. The different experiment days follow qualitatively similar behaviour, but are visibly distinct to one another, indicating again, that there are some uncontrolled parameters, that are different between these experiment days. Candidates are the

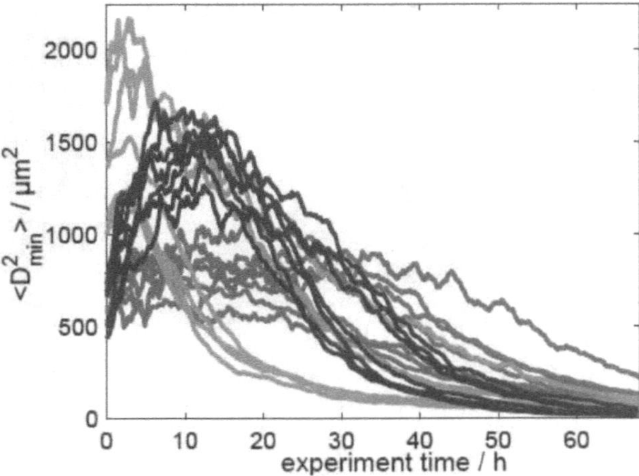

Figure 4.5: Time evolution of the mean magnitude of nonaffine displacement D^2_{min} during the next 2h after each frame of the experiments. The colours indicate sets of measurements on the same day.

initial cell density, that was varied intentionally, the exact time since passage, which varied slightly and the cell number density of the flask before passage.

The rearrangement dynamics show a 7-40 fold slow down over the experiment time of three days. The mean magnitude of nonaffine displacement does not completely vanish, even for matured layers, but goes to a value of roughly $100\,\mu m^2$, which is smaller than the typical squared radius of adherent, confluent MCF-10A cells. This means that the relative cell motion is substantially smaller than a cell size ($> 400\,\mu m^2$), which characterizes a jammed cell layer. There is no jump in the rearrangement dynamics of the cells visible, which excludes the possibility of a 'first-order like' state transition between fluid and solid behaviour. It is important to keep in mind that a jammed system is not necessarily fully arrested, because it just means that there is a yield-stress needed for cell rearrangement, which can be overcome by the intrinsic motility of cells.

There is one key distinction, that I want to point out here. Jammed-like tissue behaviour is not equivalent to a lack of cell motion, but rather to a lack of cell rearrangements within the tissue. Figure 4.6 can be considered as an illustration of this distinctions. When an epithelial layer is cultivated densely before a wound healing experiment is conducted, it will be able to invade the wound, but it will do so in collective fashion, resembling laminar flow. This is already visible in the yellow track indicators of the left image in figure 4.6. These tracks form parallel lines that seldom cross, resembling flow lines in laminar flows. This assessment is validated by the mean magnitude of nonaffine displacement of cells in the layer during the wound closure, which is plotted in the right side of figure 4.6. Most of the cell movement during the epithelial wound closure is an affine, collective motion of the whole layer. The nonaffine displacement is with a mean of maximal $70\,\mu\text{m}^2$ substantially smaller than the typical squared radius of adherent, confluent MCF-10A cells, signifying a very low amount of cell rearrangements within the layer. The difference to random fluid-like behaviour that allows for easy cell rearrangements is visible when comparing the mean magnitude of nonaffine displacement to early, sparse configurations of the layer in figure 4.2, where D^2_{min} reaches values of over $1000\,\mu\text{m}^2$.

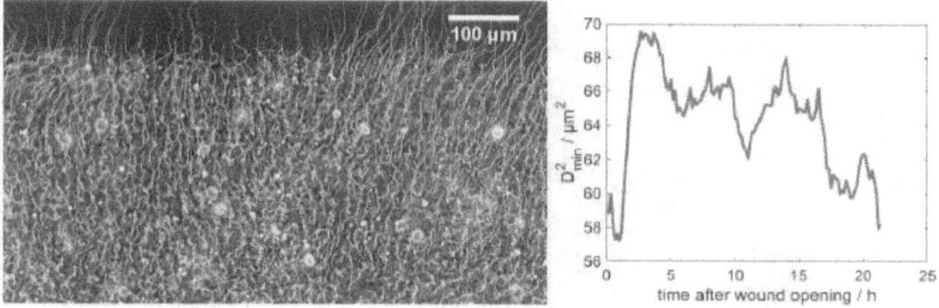

Figure 4.6: The left image depicts a MCF-10A monolayer shortly after removing a wound healing insert. The grey phase contrast image is overlaid with red fluorescence nuclei signal and yellow indications of the tracks that the cells take in the coming 5 hours. Please note that these tracks are over a longer time compared to the previous images. The right plot depicts the time-evolution of the mean magnitude of nonaffine displacement of cells in the epithelial-like layer during the wound closure.

This distinction between lack of motion and inability of rearrangements is important since the cell jamming transition is still often characterized as a change in velocity [178], and a tissue flow into cell free regions is often characterized as fluidisation [94, 186, 188]. While these categorizations are not inherently wrong, they fail to appreciate that the fundamental property of the tissue, to either enable or disable cell rearrangements, does not have to change. There is therefore a strong link between cell jamming and collective motion, since a tissue that suppresses nonaffine motion can only move in an affine, collective way. The ability to do so does not contradict a way of jamming, since the classical examples of jammed grains need solid boundary conditions to stay jammed and transmit forces to the outside. The other typical comparison, glasses, is a little more flawed in this case, as glasses can slow down their fluidity even in the absence of strong boundary conditions, which is hardly observed in cells. More considerations of the interplay between tissue dynamics and their boundaries can be found in chapter 4.2

4.1.2   Measures of glassy motion in cellular systems

There are various ways to quantify the cell dynamics within tissues. In this chapter I will discuss a part of them on the data set that was already introduced in the previous chapter, in order to compare what the individual statements mean and how the overall picture is emerging. For all these analysis, the motion of the cell nuclei, tracked using fluorescence stain, are used as a substitute for the cell movement. The focus are the measures, that can be used to quantify the cell jamming transition.

Figure 4.7 displays on of the most standard metrics of cell motion on the left side: the mean squared displacement(MSD) of the cells within a certain time period, often called lag time, plotted over this lag time. One exemplary scene of an experiment is displayed and divided into 5 consecutive time periods. It is evident that the movement within the cell layer slows down significantly over time, since the MSDs for all these consecutive time periods are ordered in descending order.

For low lag times the increase in the mean squared displacement for increasing lag times roughly follows the ballistic behaviour of $\propto \tau^2$, that is usual in this regime. There, the cell or nucleus motion is so small in magnitude and time period, that the object does not have any occasion to change its course, caused by, for example, an obstacle. For higher lag times the derivative of the mean squared displacement to the lag time is curved throughout and decreases to slightly below $\propto \tau^1$, which would be normal diffusive behaviour. This is a small indication for jammed behaviour, but alone it would be far from enough to prove it, since there is only subtle difference and the effect is not pronounced. The main reason is that even in states where cell rearrangements are inhibited, there are drifts within the layer, where groups of cells move towards

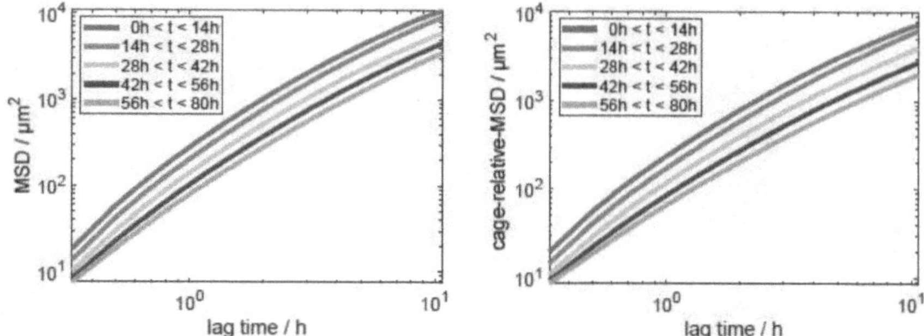

Figure 4.7: Mean squared displacement and caged mean squared displacement of the nuclei movement within 5 consecutive time periods of an exemplary scene of the experiment.

regions of lower cell number density.

The right side of figure 4.7 helps to estimate this collective behaviour. It shows the cage-relative MSD, which subtracts the mean velocity vector of the neighbouring cells from the travelled distance of the cells before the mean squared displacement is calculated. It is called cage-relative, because in classic examples of jammed systems, these neighbours build the cage for the cell in question. For small lag times the cage-relative mean squared displacement is very similar to the normal MSD and describes a ballistic-like motion as described above. For high lag times the absolute value as well as the derivative of the cage-relative mean squared displacement is the normal MSD. This is a strong sign that a large amount of the 'low-frequency' motion is collective, as the subtraction of independently moving neighbours would add an additional noise term and increase the cage-relative MSD compared to the normal MSD [197]. The sub-diffusive behaviour exhibited by the cage-relative MSD is still not very convincing, which shows another flaw of this kind of analysis: One needs to include ensembles over a very long time interval to access the behaviour for long lag times, because otherwise the fluctuations are too strong. There also should not be a lot of change within the ensemble since the inherently averaging metric of the mean squared displacements will average over these changes. These considerations explain that this measure is only useful to characterize a certain stable or quasi-stable state when it is measured long enough and not the transition between states such as a fluid and solid one, which will be described in chapter 4.3

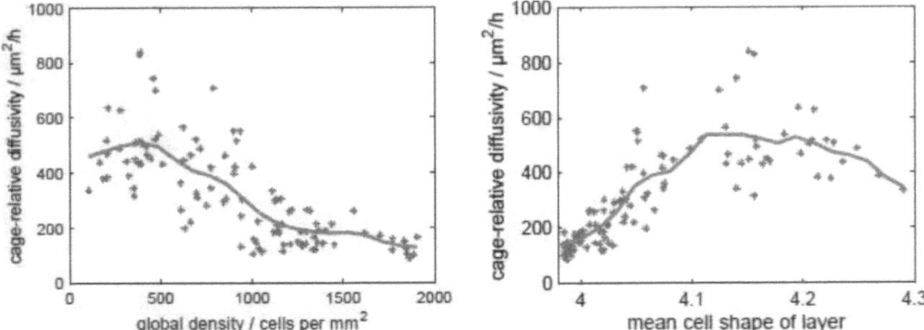

Figure 4.8: Individual experiments were divided into 5 ensembles of consecutive time periods. The cage-relative diffusivities is plotted over the mean global cell number density(left) and mean shape parameter(right) as blue dots for each ensemble. The orange curves are moving averages of the blue data point with Gaussian kernels.

Despite the flaws of the MSD approach for the study of the jamming transition, there is still knowledge to be gained from it. One can construct a measure of the amount of rearrangements out of the cage-relative MSD, even though it can only function as a mean over a large ensemble. For that purpose, all experimental scenes were divided into 5 consecutive time periods similar to figure 4.7 and a cage-relative diffusivity was estimated by dividing the cage-relative mean squared displacement at the lag time of 10 hours by mentioned 10 hours. In figure 4.9 these cage-relative diffusivities were plotted over the mean global cell number density (left) and mean shape parameter (right) of the averaged ensembles. The data points are plotted as blue dots and are averages with a Gaussian kernel as an orange guiding line. For both of the structural parameters, the measure of tissue rearrangement diminishes by a factor of about 2.5 between the peak and the minimum. The peaks at low global cell number density and high global shape parameter are associated with early times in the experiment, while the minimum is associated with late experiment times. The decrease in cage-relative diffusivity depending on an increase in global cell number density is roughly smooth and steady. In contrast, the mean cell shape has only an influence below the value of 4.1, but in this range it has a strong influence that appears to be linear. The measured shape indices are higher than predicted by the simulations of shape-induced jamming transitions with Vertex models [30, 31, 32], but before one concludes a contradiction one has to reflect, that the tessellation around nuclei tends to overestimate the cell shapes of ensembles with low shape indices. The numerical accuracy of the predicted critical shape parameter of the model of the shape-induced jamming transition is still questioned by this result.

Thus far in this chapter, I have only described measures of cell and tissue dynamic that inherently average over large ensembles. Since one of the goals of this thesis is to describe the processes during the jamming transition I require measures that have a better temporal and spatial resolution. Figure 4.9 shows some of the possible measures, as time evolution graphs, of the same data set shown previously and the different scenes coloured individually. The left graph shows the change of the mean cell velocity per hour, determined as the distance the cells move within an hour. While it signifies a marked decrease over time, there is still a large residue value in the regions that other measures describe as arrested. This background velocity stems from small scale motion of the nuclei in the cages formed by their neighbours, small collective motion events and simple detection errors. It is also important to keep in mind that this velocity does not address rearrangements directly, as discussed at the end of chapter 4.1.1. The spike near the end of the graphs stems from a medium change that lead to a small misalignment in the time series of the experiment. It is visible that the mean cell velocities increase slightly after refreshing the medium, but not drastically compared to the start of the experiment.

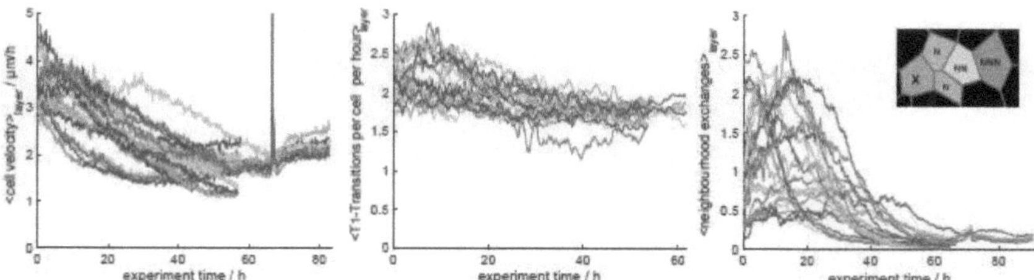

Figure 4.9:   Different estimators of the tissue dynamics, that are not inherently ensemble averages, are plotted as time evolutions over the experiment time. The left figure shows the mean cell velocity, the middle figure shows the mean amount of T1-transitions per hour and the right figure shows the mean amount of neighbourhood exchanges within the next 4 hours. A neighbourhood exchange happens when a cell receives a new neighbour that did not share a neighbour with the cell in question at the start of the time of the 4 hours. The topological distance that a cell has to traverse is indicated in the insert.

The graph in the middle of figure 4.9 depicts the time evolution of T1-transitions per hour. A T1-transition in a tessellation is occurring, when the edge between two vertices disappears and the vertex afterwards splits again building an edge in the orthogonal direction. This process changes locally which cells are neighbours of each other, is the minimal topological transition required for rearrangements and therefore often used in theory and simulations [227, 30, 228]. I measured the T1 transitions by checking in each frame for each cell if it acquired a new neighbour. Cells in whose neighbourhoods tracks disappear or appear were sorted out from the analysis. Experimentally this measure of T1 transitions is too noisy to give reliable results. In many configurations of cells, small fluctuations of the nuclei position within their cell body are enough to trigger T1-transitions. This explains, why the decrease in the in T1-transitions per hour is so small in the center part of figure 4.9.

The inability to reliably quantify topological changes experimentally with T1-transitions motivated me to develop a measure that is more robust in regards to fluctuations and experimental noise. The idea is that a system that allows rearrangements will contain cells that shift places with other cells and topologically move more than one T1-transition in a sufficiently long time period. The exact definition for such a rearrangement event, that I coined neighbourhood exchange, for any given cell ended up being the acquisition of a new neighbour that did not share a neighbour with the given cell at the start of a four hour time period. That requires at least 3 different T1 transitions and a robust amount of movement that is not obtainable by small fluctuations. Any cell pairs, whose tracks ended in the neighbourhood within the four hour time period were discarded, because it is hard to automatically check, whether that disappearance was an error and the resulting possible neighbourhood exchange an artefact. The time period of four hours turned out to be a reasonable one by checking the behaviour of the measure at different time periods, but since I will mostly use the magnitude of nonaffine displacement D_{min}^2 to quantify the rearrangement dynamics of tracked monolayers later on, I will not go into more detail about the metric of neighbourhood exchanges.

The main point is that the metric of neighbourhood exchanges, plotted on the right side of figure 4.9, inherently measures the ability of cells to rearrange in tissues. Time evolution of this measure is very similar to the time evolution of the magnitude of nonaffine displacement D_{min}^2 in figure 4.5. In the beginning, during the fluid part of the layer development, the mean amount of neighbourhood exchanges per cell within four hours reach values of about 1.5 to 2.5 and this value reduces very sharply to values between 0.05 and 0.2. Again, as for D^2_{min}, this part can be regarded as jammed since the rearrangements are drastically slowed down and even in a jammed system active particles with appropriate energy can overcome energy barriers. There are potentially experts that would only characterize a fully arrested system as jammed and call the one described here partially jammed, but I view this discussion as a little semantic and do not plan to indulge in it. Similar to the leftmost plot in figure 4.9, depicting the velocity development, there is an artefact introduced near the end of the time evolution by a change of medium. Similarly, the amount of neighbourhood exchanges recovers slightly with fresh medium, but stays at a drastically lower value than in the fluid regime at the beginning of the experiment. This will be important later in the discussion of the influence of an ageing effect on the rearrangement dynamics in the system.

4.1.3   Biophysical changes during jamming transition

The characterization in the two previous chapters shows that the system of epithelial-like MCF-10A cells behaves fluid like for low densities and shortly after it grows confluent, but exhibits a transition into a dynamic arrest shortly after confluency. This is more deeply discussed in the chapter 4.3, but here I would like to focus on the cell biological changes that are connected with jamming transition. From a biophysical point of view the main candidates are: cell adhesion, contractility, cell stiffness.

Here, I employ fluorescence images of molecular components in the different dynamic stages to study how the biophysical components in the system evolve. I received help with the fluorescence images from Carlotta Ficorella. MCF-10A layers were seeded and observed with phase contrast microscopy to confirm that dynamic behaviour of the cell layers that were later stained was similar to the cell layers that were tracked for the analysis presented in the previous chapters.

Typical images of desmosomes (green) and cytokeratin (red) of MCF-10A layers after 1-3 days of development are shown in figure 4.10. Some of the boarders between cells are bright lines in the desmoplakin signal, but by far not all of them, which can be double checked by looking at the nuclei (blue) as a measure of the amount of cells. This stands in contrast to the images of e-cadherin in figure 4.11, where most cell boundaries were visible. However, it is consistent with other published work, where MCF-10A cells exhibit less pronounced desmosomes than other epithelial cell lines

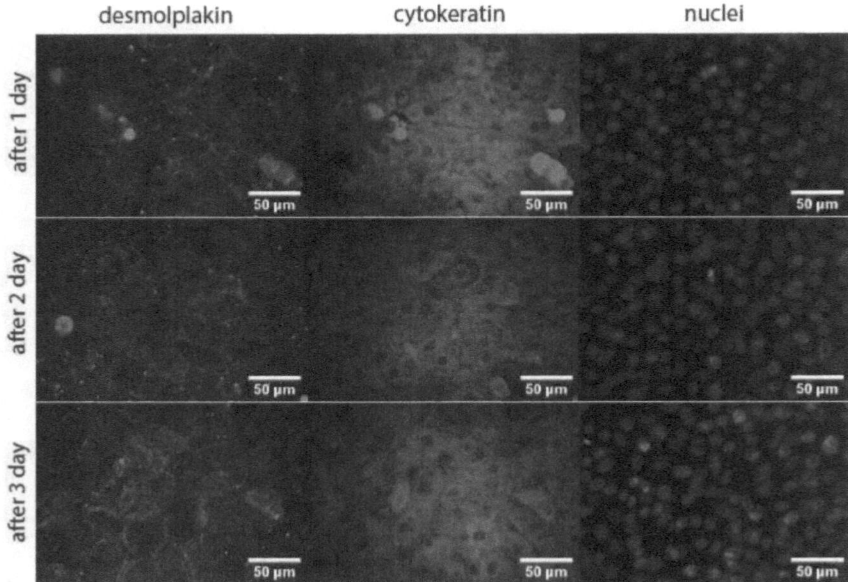

Figure 4.10: Desmosomes, cytokeratin and nuclei of cell layers fixed and stained after consecutive days of development. The rows correspond to the days the layer was allowed to develop corresonding to the time of the tracking experiment. The column show the stained desmosomes, cytokeratin and nuclei of the layer in this order from left to right.

[229, 230]. The keratin signal is homogeneously distributed besides a decrease at some boundaries and nuclei. One might think that the abundance of nuclei compared to visible boundaries indicates additional layers of cells, but no further desmoplakin or keratin structures are visible by shifting trough the z-space. The structures are barely visible and do not change much over time, which gives strong indications that they are not a driving factor of the solidification that occurs during the time between the first and the third day of the experiment.

Figure 4.11 shows the E-cadherin stain of layers from day 1 to day 3 in the bottom column with the corresponding actin stain in the top column. Since, E-cadherin, one of the major markers of epithelial cells, gets down regulated during the development of carcinoma and is connected with signalling pathways within the cell, it is one of

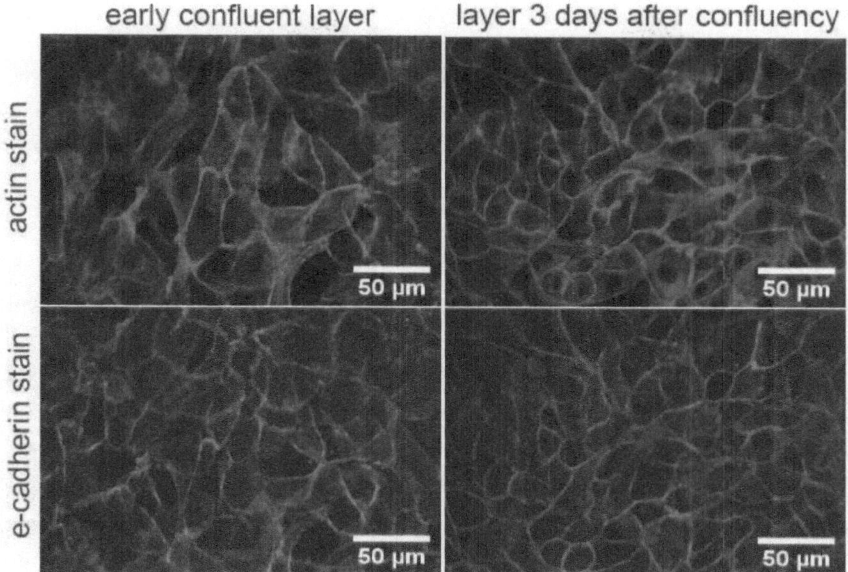

Figure 4.11: MCF-10A cell layer were cultivated until certain points in their develop and fixed and stained afterwards. In the top column fluorescence stains of the f-actin cytoskeleton are shown in red and E-cadherin is shown in green in the bottom column. The left row depicts an exemplary region from a one-day old, motile cell layer while the right row depicts a three-day old nearly arrested cell layer.

the suspects for controlling the dynamic behaviour [231, 232, 38, 34]. This thesis does indeed contain strong evidence, that the down regulation of E-cadherin can induce unjamming as shown later in chapter 4.2, but judging from figure 4.11 it is not the only driving factor of the jamming transition. Similar to the desmosome images in figure 4.10, there are no striking differences in the E-cadherin intensity between fluorescence images of layers from day 1 to day 3, whereas the rearrangement dynamics changes strongly similar to figure 4.5. The observed structures were also qualitatively similar, whereby the cell boundaries are noticeably less fluctuating at later stages. These are strong indications that the dynamical slow-down is NOT a maturing of cell adhesion bounds, as it was previously reported for a very similar system by Garcia et al. [27].

The most visible bio-mechanical changes were connected to the actin cytoskeleton.

Actin stress fibers are ever visible after the first day of the experiment and not at later times (fig 4.11 top). This is consistent with a recent report that identified a decrease in traction as one of the driving factors of cell jamming [190]. At later times, the most prominent actin structures are the cortices, which are again, visibly straighten up over time. I initially interpreted this straightening as a sign of increasing cortex tension, which motivated optical stretcher measurements to examine this line of thinking. I received help with the those from Hannah-Marie Scholz-Marggraf.

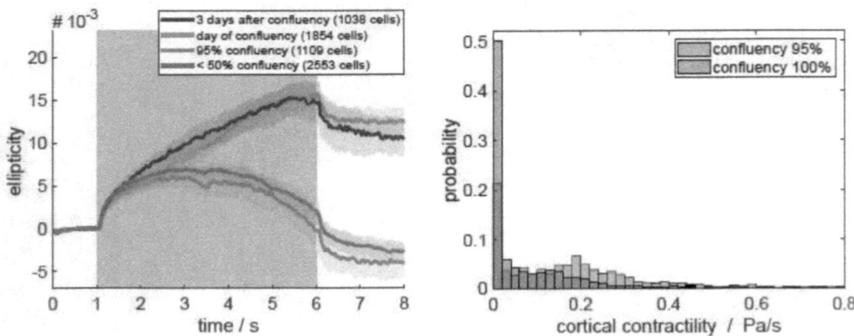

Figure 4.12:   The plot on the left side depicts deformation of MCF-10A cells under stress in optical stretcher experiments. These cells were cultured up to differing points of volume fraction and cell number density, than detached and measured. Especially for sparse cells an increasing resistance to the outside stress is visible, since a decrease in relative deformation under continued stress is not describable as a passive viscoelastic material. The right graph shows a histogram of the fitted values of cortical contractility for the measured cells.

For these measurements, MCF-10A cells were cultivated up to different densities, corresponding to different dynamical states of the system and than detached. The optical stretcher set-up measures deformations of cells in suspension caused by the optical force of two lasers [233, 234]. During the 5 second stretch shown in the left part of figure 4.12, the measured cells can contract against the out-side force using their actomyosin machinery [205, 206]. This can lead to a decrease in the visible strain against the out-side stress, that is not explainable by a non-active viscoelastic material. The behaviour is fitted well by the extended Kelvin-Voigt model, that is one of the most frequently used models for passive cell deformation plus a tension that is increasing linearly in time, thus motivating the description of a contractility in Pa/s. Histograms of the estimated contractilities for the measured cells are shown in the right part of figure 4.12. The contractility is attributable to the actomyosin machinery in the actin cortex, since cells lose their stress fibres in suspension [235], and the effect can be suppressed with blebbistatin [206]. Contrary to our initial expectation, cells that were extracted from dense, confluent layers had a median cortical contractility of about 0.09 Pa/s which is halve of the value of cells that were not confluent, which is 0.18 Pa/s. This finding does however conform well to other published results, such as the fact that the traction inside epithelial tissues is low compared to boarder regions, where pronounced rims can be formed [87, 236]. The most surprising facet of this data, is that the change in cortical contractility seems sharply occurring while the cell layer reaches confluence. One possible explanation is that a large amount of the traction in epithelial cell layers is generated by the border cells, as previously reported by [237, 238]. The inner cells build "floating islands" that do not exhibit much traction and are compressed by the boarder cells. The loss of the boarder cells when the cell layer reaches confluence could trigger a change in phenotype.

The decrease of cortical contractility should push cells to higher cell shapes and is therefore counter-intuitive with the jamming transition and the SPV model in mind. First of all, this change seems to occur directly when the layer becomes confluent, where most of the layers observed in the previous chapter are still decently motile. It is also not the only factor driving the development of the epithelial layer. In the tracking experiments, I observed a tendency to rounder cell shapes with the estimation using the Voronoi-tessellation as seen in figure 4.2. The lowering of cortical contractility seems to be compensated by, for example, the disappearance of actin stress fibres. Even the lower cortical contractility of densely packed epithelial cells is higher than the cortical contractility of mesenchymal-like cells [206].

For the influence on cell jamming the most important finding here is that a change in cell-cell adhesion is not necessary, for the collective arrest in motion and that this arrest coincides with a change of the F-actin structure from an inherently asymmetric stress fibre structure to a more symmetric cortex pattern. This changes the stresses that cells tend to evoke from an anisotropic profile, that is connected to motility and allows for many degrees of freedom on a tissue level to an isotropic profile on the level of cells connected to a lower intrinsic velocity, rounder cells and less degrees of freedom for cell motion on a tissue level.

At the start of this chapter I mentioned cell stiffness as a possible changing biophysical cell parameter, that might be connected with the jamming transition. At first glance the fluorescence images of the cytoskeleton do not give rise to the assumption that the stiffness is increasing, as the intensity stay similar and, beside the loss of actin stress fibres, the architecture of the structures does not change drastically. The parameters characterizing the viscoelastic response of the detached cells in the optical stretcher measurements of figure 4.12 are also relatively stable and form no basis for a conjecture of an increasing cell stiffness. Even with these findings in mind, I would not rule out that an increasing effective cell stiffness plays at least a minor role during the cell jamming transition since the transition is accompanied by an increase in cell number density and a compression of the individual cells and biological materials often stiffen under compression [239]. This is just a conjecture at this point and needs to be studied, but it is an interesting starting point to explain the strong role of cell number density on the rearrangement dynamics that will be discussed in chapter 4.3.

4.2   Tissue fluidity in the context of ECM boundaries

Cancer metastasis is the most prominent and important occasion, where a change in the ability of cells to move has disastrous consequences. This process is currently the focus of scientific research, since a comprehensive understanding of it would allow to better prognosticate and possibly treat cancer patients saving potentially millions of lives. One of the major cell biological changes that cancer metastasis is connected with is the epithelial-mesenchymal transition (EMT) [34]. Within the EMT the loss or down regulation of the adhesion molecule E-cadherin is thought to be a key contributor to the changing phenotype, since the molecule is connected to many signalling pathways within the cell. While there is a large amount of literature about E-cadherin from a cell biological perspective, there is less known on the effect of E-cadherin down regulation on the tissue dynamics [181]. I was involved in a cooperation with the group of Prof. Friedl investigating this question. They did perform the experiments and biological alterations on the cells, while I did cell tracking in the motility experiments, segmentation of the cells and the analysis of both. While I will focus on my results in this chapter I obviously have to mention some of the other results of this cooperation in order to explain and interpret my results. The core of this work has been published in Nature Cell Biology [33].

4.2.1   Down regulation of E-cadherin elongates cells

The experiments I analysed were done using 4T1 cell lines, which is a cancer cell line that is classified as highly invasive and metastatic, but still expresses E-cadherin [43, 44]. Two phenotypes based on this cell line were prepared by the group of Prof. Friedl: The shCDH1 phenotype had a stable down regulation of the gene expression of CDH1, which encodes E-cadherin, of about 85%-95%, while the shNT phenotype served as control and had to endured the same procedure but no genes were targeted [33]. The abbreviation NT stands for non targeted. I will also use the expressions E-cadherin^{low} and E-cadherin^{high} for these two phenotypes.

I will start by describing the morphological changes that were caused by the down regulation of E-cadherin in the 4T1 cell line, since those will inform the discussion of changes in the tissue dynamics. Spheroids of the two cell types were seeded on the bottom of a petri dish and embedded into a 2 mg/ml collagen network, that was used as proxy for the extracellular matrix. Those spheroids were granted 48 hours to expand into and invade the collagen network. Afterwards, they were fixed, stained and imaged with a laser scanning microscope. I analysed these images with a self-written Matlab algorithm, which is described in chapter 3.0.2 to produce a two-dimensional cell segmentation in order to estimate the properties of the tissue structure.

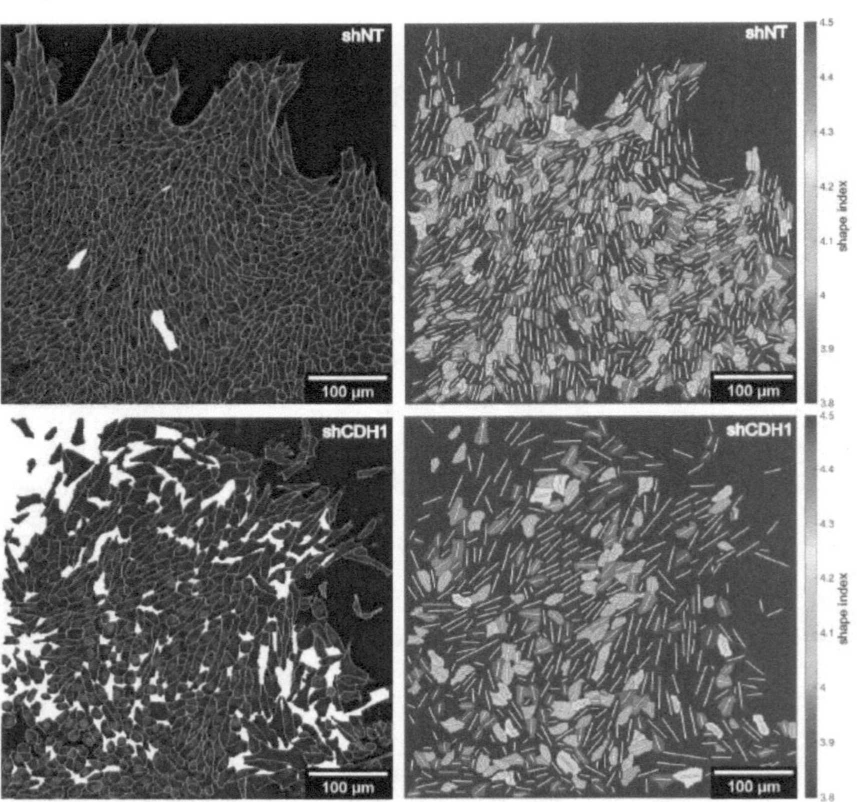

Figure 4.13: The right column depicts spheroids of shNT(top) and shCDH1(bottom) cells expanding into 2 mg/ml collagen. The F-actin fluorescence signal is coloured green, the nucleus flourescence signal is coloured red and the white lines form the borders of cells estimated by a cell segmentation. White areas overlay cell free regions inside a spheroid. The right column pictures the segmented cell areas colour coded with the shape index of the segments. The white lines are indicators of the cell orientation.

The left column of figure 4.13 shows example images of the structure of E-cadherin^{high} and E-cadherin^{low} spheroids invading 2 mg/ml collagen networks on a petri dish. The green colour signifies the fluorescence signal of F-actin; the red colour is depicting the nuclei and the white outlines show the borders between the segmented cells. White areas within the tissue represent a cell-free region within the spheroid. A visualization of the structural features is on the right side of the figure. The shape indices of the segmented cells are colour coded and there are lines in the direction of the longest axis of the corresponding second moment tensor to indicate the orientation of the cells.

The clearest observation that arises from figure 4.13 is that the down regulation of E-cadherin leads to a loss of cohesion in the spheroid structure. There are drastically more cell free regions in the spheroid of E-cadherin^{low} cells and they lack the cohesion of the E-cadherin^{high} cells. These cell free regions in E-cadherin^{low} spheroids mean, that these spheroids have a volume fraction lower than one, in contrast to most other systems discussed in this thesis. There are individual E-cadherin^{low} cells that invade the collagen, which is not the case for E-cadherin^{high}. Those have a clear boundary to the collagen network and finger-like protrusions. The cells near the tips of the protrusions often probe the environment with lamellipodia-like structures, resembling leader cells in epithelial monolayers. The E-cadherin^{high} spheroid gives the impression of having a surface tension, because the boundary is very smooth even at the points where the cells that form the boarder, change. Additionally, some cells between the protrusions elongate and orientate along the boundaries. E-cadherin^{low} spheroids lack such a clear boundary. It is sometimes even hard in to define, where the spheroid ends and where the region with individually invading cells start.

The E-cadherin^{low} cells are on average more elongated than E-cadherin^{high} cells, which is indicated by the increasing amount of dark red coloured cells in the lower right of figure 4.13. There are more extremely elongated cells. Both of these cell types are significantly above the critical shape index of the SPV model, which is at 3.814. A visual inspection gives the impression, that elongated cells tend to have elongated nuclei. This is not analysed and proven here, but it will be interesting to keep in mind, as this is a more central point in the analysis of a similar system later in the thesis. It is very apparent, that E-cadherin^{high} cells are packed more densely in the spheroid than the E-cadherin^{low} low cells, in both possible meanings of density; the volume fraction of cells and their number density. The orientation of the cells in both cell types tends to point to the outside of the spheroids, which is to be expected, while the cells are in the process of invading the ECM.

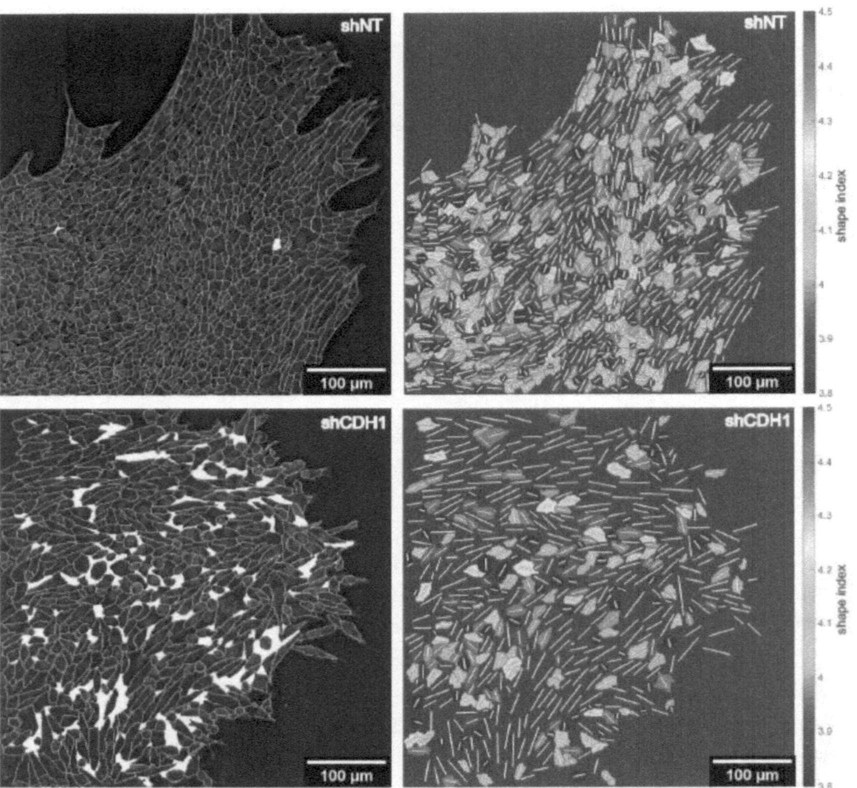

Figure 4.14: The right column depicts spheroids of shNT(top) and shCDH1(bottom) cells expanding into 6 mg/ml collagen. The F-actin fluorescence signal is coloured green, the nucleus flourescence signal is coloured red and the white lines form the borders of cells estimated by a cell segmentation. White areas overlay cell free regions inside a spheroid. The right column pictures the segmented cell areas colour coded with the shape index of the segments. The white lines are indicators of the cell orientation. [33]

The lines indicating the cell orientation in the right column of figure 4.13 suggest, that the cells, especially E-cadherin^{high} cells, have a very high alignment in the orientation with their local environment. This bears true, when examining this behaviour with a two-dimensional nematic order parameter. Thereby the director is always a particular cell and the angle of the orientation with its neighbours is used for the local nematic order parameter. E-cadherin^{high} cells reach a value of about 0.44, while the value of E-cadherin^{low} cells is 0.39. These values incorporate 3 spheroids each for collagen networks with density 2 and 6 mg/ml. Although the numerical values are in the range associated with nematic phases, this is not a fully nematic order because the order parameter is too low and even more so because the director is defined locally. Nevertheless, there is still a significant orientational correlation within the tissue structure. The orientational alignment likely has multiple causes, ranging from Onsagers arguments about the entropy in the ordering of elongated particles, to cell polarization and elongation in the direction of movement, which has a bias outwards of the spheroid, to possibly Vicsek-like polar alignment, that postulates that adhering cells tend to move in the same direction [195]. The fact that E-cadherin^{low} cells are less aligned seems logical given the additional degrees of freedom due to the open spaces inside the spheroid. Interestingly, the local nematic order parameters for the outside regions are considerably higher than those for the inside regions (E-cadherin$^{high}_{outside}$: S= 0.46; E-cadherin$^{high}_{inside}$: S= 0.39), underlining the suspicion, that the motion into the collagen region is at least partially responsible for the alignment.

Figure 4.14 shows the same content as figure 4.13 except that the spheroids are embedded in collagen network with a density of 6 mg/ml. Most of the structural features and differences of E-cadherin^{high} and E-cadherin^{low} spheroids in 6 mg/ml collagen networks are very similar to those spheroids in 2 mg/ml collagen networks. I will not repeat all the properties and mostly focus on those that change. It is apparent, that the E-cadherin^{low} do not invade the denser collagen network individually. Importantly, even in these condensed conditions the E-cadherin^{low} cells are individualized and non-cohesive in the spheroid. The local orientation correlation of the E-cadherin^{low} cells is a little higher for the spheroids embedded in the 6 mg/ml collagen networks than in the 2 mg/ml collagen networks, probably because the cells are packed more densely and the steric effects are stronger. The E-cadherin^{high} cells tend to be a little rounder in the spheroids in higher density networks, especially in the center region, which indicates that the elongation of these cells is connected with their motion.

Two aspects of the numerical analysis of the cell shapes are plotted in figure 4.15. The left part of that figure shows the distribution of the aspect ratios of the segmented cell shapes of E-cadherin^{high} and E-cadherin^{low} spheroids in the boarder regions with 6 mg/ml collagen network. It is apparent, that the distribution of cell elongations is

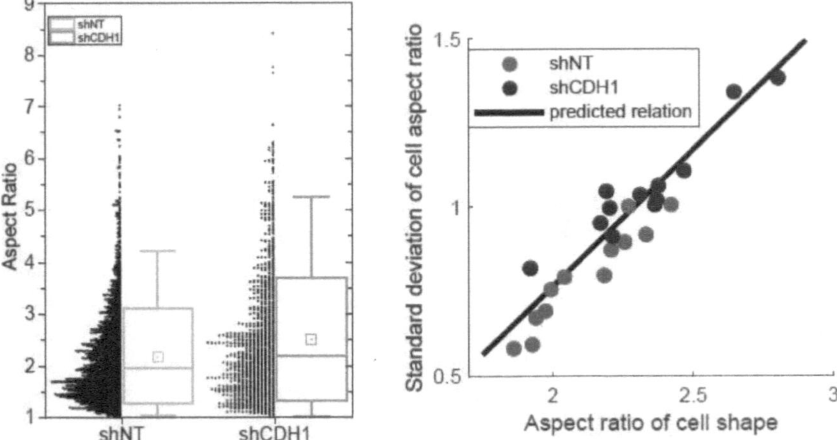

Figure 4.15: The left figure shows the distribution of cell elongations in the boarder regions of E-cadherin^{high} 4T1/shNT spheroids and E-cadherin^{low} 4T1/shCDH1 spheroids in 6 mg/ml collagen networks at the bottom of petri dishes. The black dots represent individual cells and the boxplot indicate the quartiles, the median with lines and the mean value with a square. The right plot shows mean values of the standard deviation of the aspect ratio plotted over the aspect ratio of the cells averaged for the middle and boarder regions of shNT and shCDH1 spheroids in both 2 and 6 mg/ml collagen networks. The black line is a predicted relation based on geometrical contraints [179] and not a fit of the data. [33]

broader for E-cadherin^{low} cells meaning there are more elongated cells, in the cell type with down regulated E-cadherin. This results also in a higher mean and median value of the aspect ratio. This is not a cherry picked example. The E-cadherin^{low} cells are generally more elongated than their non-targeted brethren.

The right graph of figure 4.15 shows a graph that connects the broadness of the distribution of cell elongations with its mean. The data are mean values of the standard deviation of the aspect ratio plotted over the aspect ratio of the cells averaged for the middle and boarder regions of shNT and shCDH1 spheroids in both 2 and 6 mg/ml collagen networks. These different conditions are not indicated in order to simplify the graph. It was first proposed by Aste and Di Matteo for granular material and adapted by Atia et al. for confluent amorphous cellular systems, that the standard deviation of the cell aspect ratio has a linear relation with the mean aspect ratio [184, 179]. The predicted relation is plotted as a black line in the right graph of figure 4.15. This is not a fit of the data. It is not trivial, that the finding of Atia et al. is transferable to this system. Firstly, it is clear that a non amorphous system, like a fully nematic system would not need to hold this relation. As discussed above the spheroids show signs of local nematic-like ordering, but they are apparently not strong enough to drive it away from the geometric constraints that underlie the predicted relation. An additional factor that makes it more surprising, that the relation between the width of the aspect ratio distribution and the mean aspect ratio holds in this system, is the existence of cell free regions within the spheroid, especially the E-cadherin^{low} spheroids. This should enable the cells to adopt their preferred cell shape more freely with less geometrical constraints. The fact, that this relation still holds indicates, that either the effect of geometrical constraints is very robust, or that these cells adopt similar cell shape distributions on their own accord without being forced by geometric constraints.

Figure 4.16 shows the distribution of segmented cell sizes for the different experimental

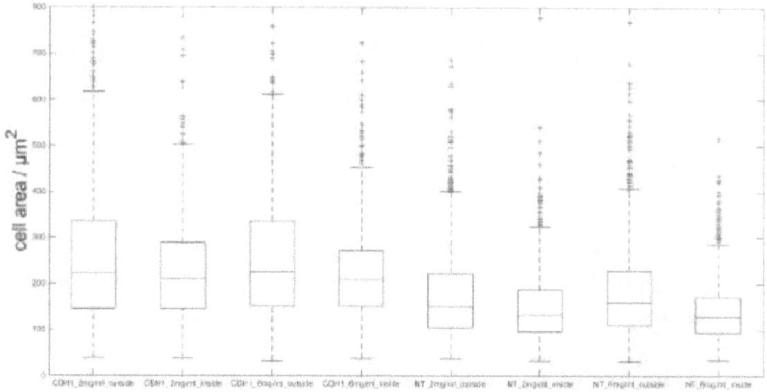

Figure 4.16: The figure shows the distribution of cell areas E-cadherin^{high} 4T1/shNT spheroids and E-cadherin^{low} 4T1/shCDH1 spheroids subdivided into different spheroid regions and different collagen network densities. The red lines show the median value of the distribution, boxes indicate the 25th and 75th percentiles and the whiskers extend to the data points within the $\pm 2.7\,\sigma$, which is the regime that is not considered outliers, by the standard Matlab algorithm. Those outliers are marked with red crosses.

conditions subdivided into the inner spheroid region and the boarder region. Keep in mind, that the mean measured cell area is roughly inverse to the cell number density of the system. The plots prove the visual impression, that the E-cadherin^{low} spheroids are drastically less packed. It is interesting, that the density of the surrounding collagen network does not have an impact on the mean cell number density in either phenotype. For both cell types the inside is a denser than the edge region, but this effect is considerably more drastic in the E-cadherin^{high} phenotype.

4.2.2 Down regulation of E-cadherin fluidizes cells

Besides the structural changes caused by the down regulation of E-cadherin, the changes in the kind of cell motion that is occurring was the focus of this study. Figure 4.17 depicts an exemplary excerpt of a motility assay, where the spheroids were put on petri dishes, embedded in collagen networks and imaged while the expand into and invade the collagen. These experiments aim to imitate the motion of cells in three-dimensional system in the region of a two-dimensional boarder. The cell movement was tracked via their nuclei in the plane of the petri dish using TrackMate as described in chapter 3.0.1 [207]. The fluorescence signal of the nuclei is visible in gray in the background and yellow track indications with time length of $\pm 2\,\text{h}$ as well as purple circles indicating the detected nuclei are overlaid. These particular images show the process of the spheroid 6 hours after seeding in 6 mg/ml collagen networks.

Already in these exemplary images there is a systematic difference visible between E-cadherin down regulated 4T1 cells and their non-targeted counterparts, which will be confirmed by analysis later on. The E-cadherin^{high} 4T1/shNT on the left side of figure 4.17 have track indicators that barely cross each other, often run in parallel and stay decently straight in a significant amount of cases. These tracks resemble those of epithelial layer closing a wound like in figure 4.6 in the chapter 4.1.1. It is important to note, that the invasion of the collagen network, that is indicated in this image does not continue unimpeded for the experiment duration. The cell group reaches regions, where the collagen network seems to stop it and provokes an arrest or reorientation. This is already visible in the top region of the spheroid and happens quicker in denser networks.

In contrast, the E-cadherin^{low} 4T1/shCDH1 cells have tracks whose indicating lines look disorganized because they often cross each other and do not stay parallel or even

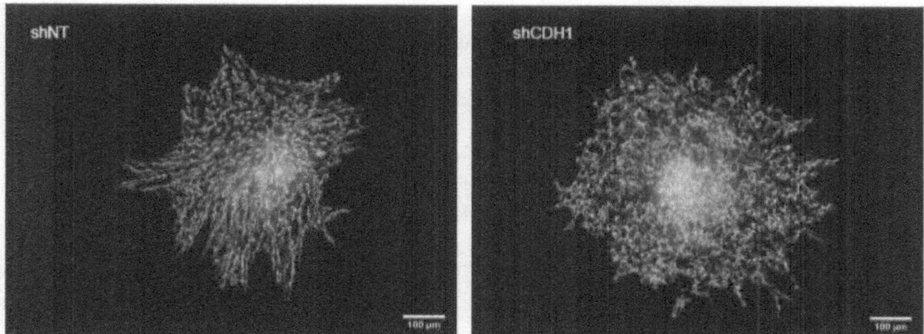

Figure 4.17: Example images of cell motility in spheroids of E-cadherin^{high} 4T1/shNT and E-cadherin^{low} 4T1/shCDH1 cells, placed on a petri dish and embedded in 6 mg/ml collagen networks. The fluorescence signal of nuclei is coloured in grey and overlaid with pink markers for detected cells and yellow indications of the tracked cell movement with a length of ± 2 h. The image is taken 6 hours after the spheroids were seeded and part of a time series, that was used to track the cells. [33]

straight. Cells regularly individualize and invade the collagen on their own, especially in sparser networks. It also occurs regularly, that cells disappear into an upper z-plane, which virtually does not happen for the E-cadherin^{high} cells. The E-cadherin^{low} cells spread wider in sparser collagen networks, but the characteristic of the movement is similar.

For the experiment that is shown in figure 4.17 and explained above, 10 spheroids in 2 independent experiments for each cell phenotype in both densities of the collagen networks were imaged by the group of Prof. Friedl and analysed by me. In some of these upcoming graphs, the tracks of each conditions were divided into the core, expanse and edge region. The core region was defined as the tracks within a 100 µm radius of the spheroid center, and the edge was defined as the 10% outermost cells. All other tracks were considered as being in the expanse. In the graphs, the E-cadherin^{high}, 4T1/shNT are coloured between green and brown/yellow while the E-cadherin^{low} 4T1/shCDH1 are coloured between blue and violet. Both are coloured more red the further away from the center the tracks are and darker in denser collagen networks.

In figure 4.18 the mean square displacements of the tracked nuclei in the analysed spheroid experiments are shown. The left graph shows the MSD's subdivided into the different spheroid regions and experimental conditions. The main difference is

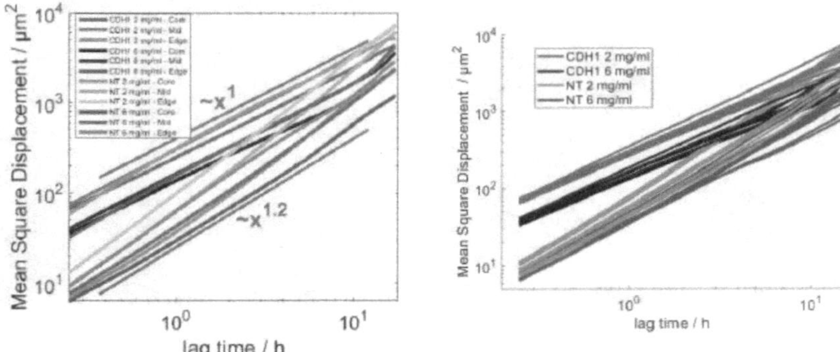

Figure 4.18: Mean squared displacements of 4T1/shNT and 4T1/shCDH1 spheroids expanding into 2 and 6 mg/ml collagen networks on a petri dish. The left graph shows the data cut into the different regions, while the right graph shows the 40 individual spheroids colour coded by cell phenotype and collagen density. [33]

that the E-cadherin^{high} behave in a superdiffusive manner and the E-cadherin^{low} cells follow a normal diffusive behaviour. The exponent of the MSD of E-cadherin^{high} cells becomes higher the more on the outside the cell tracks are and the lower the collagen density is, but it is always above 1.2 during the experiment time period. One can attribute the superdiffusive behaviour to the collective, persistent type of cell motion, that was already indicated in the parallel straight tracks and is verified below. There is a directed, collective motion from the spheroid center into the open space, similar to epithelial tissue during wound closure [85, 196]. For E-cadherin^{low} cells, the only difference between the experiment conditions is that cell velocity is higher in spheroids embedded in less dense collagen networks. Since the cells show a normal diffusive behaviour for all experiment conditions this difference in the velocity shifts the whole MSD plot upwards. The right graph in figure 4.18 depicts the MSD's for the analysed spheroids individually combining the different regions, coloured according to the cell phenotype and collagen density. The differences in the behaviour of the cells for the different experiment conditions are reproduced, when averaging over all regions. The plotted cellular behaviour is consistent between experiments, visualised by the small spread of lines of the same conditions.

The spatial and temporal velocity correlations of the tracked nuclei within spheroids expanding into collagen networks are shown in figure 4.19. For the spatial velocity

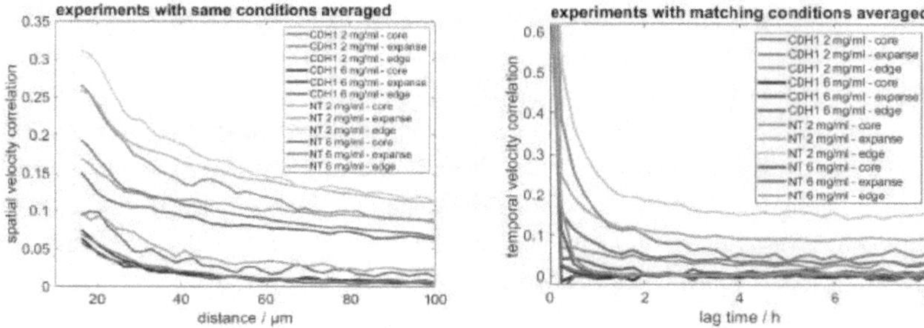

Figure 4.19: Spatial (left) and temporal (right) velocity correlation graphs of the nuclei movement in the experiments described above. The data is subdivided into the different experiment conditions and spheroid regions. The velocity correlations are estimated using Pearson correlations and smoothed with a Gaussian kernel. [33]

correlation function, the velocity correlations between close-by cells at the same time were estimated by Pearson correlations and ordered according to their distance in space. The cloud of data points was afterwards averaged with a Gaussian kernel. The plots of the spatial velocity start at distance between nuclei of $18\,\mu m$ because there is an additional effect at lower distances of cells pushing each other away, that would overcomplicate the graph. Analogously for the temporal velocity correlation function, the velocity correlation between the movements of the same cells at close-by times were estimated by Pearson correlations and ordered according to their distance in time, followed by Gaussian averaging.

It is very apparent in these graphs, that the E-cadherin^{low} cells have nearly no temporal velocity correlation and only a very minute spatial velocity correlation. This small spatial correlation is presumably caused by the asymmetry of the system promoting the cells to slightly bias their movement outwards of the densely packed spheroid. This lack of collective or persistent movement, together with the exponent of one shown in the MSD provides a clear picture of individual, fluid-like, diffusive behaviour for the E-cadherin^{low} cells.

In contrast to the E-cadherin^{low} cells, their non-targeted E-cadherin^{high} brethren display a pronounced spatial and temporal velocity correlation. The correlations are lowest for the core region of spheroids embedded in 6 mg/ml collagen gel and increase for regions closer to the boarder of the spheroids and for sparser 2 mg/ml collagen networks. These spatial and temporal velocity correlations verify a collective and persistent cell motion, that was already signified by the parallel nature of the cell tracks and the superdiffusive exponent of the MSD. These considerations explain, why the strength of the correlations is higher in regions and conditions that allow for a more pronounced collective movement. Together, these findings do not paint a picture of freely moving E-cadherin^{high} cells and suggest that they move together with their neighbours and thus behave more like an epithelial layer that has a direction it can expand into, similar to the cell behaviour in figure 4.6.

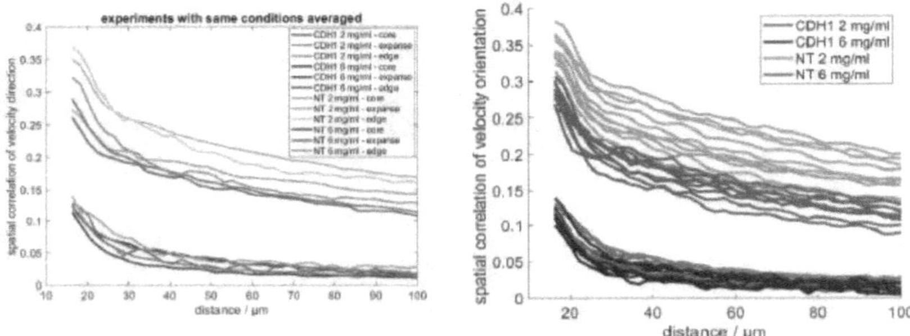

Figure 4.20: Spatial correlation of the velocity orientation of the nuclei movement in the experiments described above. The correlations are estimated using Pearson correlations and smoothed with a Gaussian kernel. The left graph shows the 40 individual spheroids colour coded by cell phenotype and collagen density. In the right graph, the data is subdivided into the different experiment conditions and spheroid regions. [33]

The graphs of the spatial correlations of the direction in which the cells move, in figure 4.20, verify all the major statements about the previous figure. The difference between E-cadherin^{high} and E-cadherin^{low} cells is a little more pronounced here, because the magnitude of the velocity introduces noise that lowers the higher correlations more. The graph on the left side of figure 4.20 depicts the individual curves of the spatial correlation of the velocity direction coloured by the cell phenotype and collagen density, and shows nearly no spread for the non-correlated E-cadherin^{low} cells, but an appreciable spread for the E-cadherin^{high} spheroids. In order to understand this, one should consider, that this correlation relates the collective movement of cells to the individual cell movement of nuclei compared to their neighbours. These fluctuations or rearrangements should be decently independent to the experimental conditions, but the collective motion is dependent on how well the cells can expand into the collagen network, where the exact local configuration of the network, which is not controllable from experiment to experiment, is a significant factor.

At this point, I would like to summarize the changes caused by the down regulation of E-cadherin. The structural images and cell segmentation show a loss of cohesion, a reduction in the packing density and an increasing cell elongation in the E-cadherin^{low} phenotype, which allows for invasion of the collagen network by individual cells. This corresponds to a shift from cohesive, collective and persistent cell movement for E-cadherin^{high} cells to individual, diffusive and fluid-like motion. It is intuitively clear that a loss of cohesion and reduction in cell density, the introduction of more free space and the increase of cell elongation allows for more degrees of freedom and fluidizes the system. Importantly, this is not what the currently most prominent theory of cell jamming, which is used in other parts of this thesis, the SPV model would have predicted on the surface [31, 32]. The Hamiltonian, that builds the foundation of this theory would have associated a decrease in adhesion, like the down regulation of a prominent adhesion molecule, with a tendency of cells to round up (instead of elongation), leading to a solidification of the system. The down regulation of E-cadherin is connected with a cascade of other cellular changes during the EMT [240] and some of those can conceivably be triggered by an artificial down regulation of E-cadherin, which could explain the shape change consistent with the SPV model. On the other hand, the model explicitly works only for confluent tissue and the loss of cohesion by down regulation of E-cadherin drives the system out of the range that is simulated by the model. This means that only a certain range of adhesions are validly described by the model and while it can give a good account what drives the jamming of cellular tissue, it can not cover the fluidisation that is occurring here. The classical concept of unjamming transition by a reduction in density, that comes from granular materials, also fits the data qualitatively. This reinforces my view, that a complete theory of biological jamming and unjamming has to include density and cohesion effects.

It is important to point out, that there sometimes is a difference in the description of collective motion and individualisation between biologists and physicists. Biologists typically accept the motion of multiple cells in a confined space as collective motion and require the spatial separation of cells from the original cluster as cell individualisation. This means that even the E-cadherin^{low} phenotype can be confined by a network dense enough, to appear collective and non-individual from a biological perspective, while the physical description does not change and the cells move individually and uncoordinated.

From a physicist point of view, one can describe the cell individualisation, that the biologist mean as a decondensation. It can only occur when the inter-particle adhesion is low enough, in this case caused by a down regulation of E-cadherin^{low}. In this analogy, the density of the collagen corresponds to the outside pressure, that can also keep the system from evaporating if it is high enough.

4.2.3 Replication of the dynamical behaviour *in vivo*

The dynamical behaviour, that the E-cadherin^{high} and E-cadherin^{low} cell spheroids exhibited *in vitro*, was verified by *in vivo* experiments. The group of Prof. Friedl implanted spheroids of both cell phenotypes, transfected with a nucleus stain, into the mammary fat pad of living mice and imaged it using multiphoton microscopy [33]. I received a time series of 3D stacks, registered them and tracked the nuclei movement in 3D using TrackMate as described in chapter 3.0.1 [207]. As far as I am aware, this is the first time that cancer cells were tracked automatically *in vivo*.

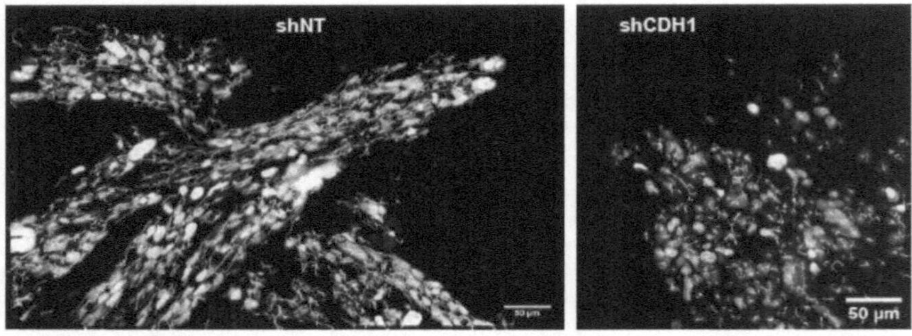

Figure 4.21: Z-projections of E-cadherin^{high} and E-cadherin^{low} cells implanted into the mammary fat pad of living mice. The nuclei are shown in grey and the 3D tracking is indicated as a projection of the indicating lines in yellow.

Figure 4.21 shows example z-projections of these implanted spheroids in living mice with fluorescent nuclei in gray and yellow track indications. The track indications are also z-trojections of three-dimensional tracks. The general tendencies of the two phenotypes of cells, that were observed *in vitro* are recovered in *in vivo*. The E-cadherin^{high} cells tend to move in clusters and the tracks tend to be parallel and straight, indicating collective and persistent motion, while the E-cadherin^{low} cells move individually and not persistent. In these experiments, many of the E-cadherin^{low} cells have a very low velocity and many seem stuck. Because of the low amount of data, owed to the complexity and required effort of the experiments, I do not feel confident to decide whether the 4T1/shCDH1 cell tend to get stuck in this environment or if this is coincidence.

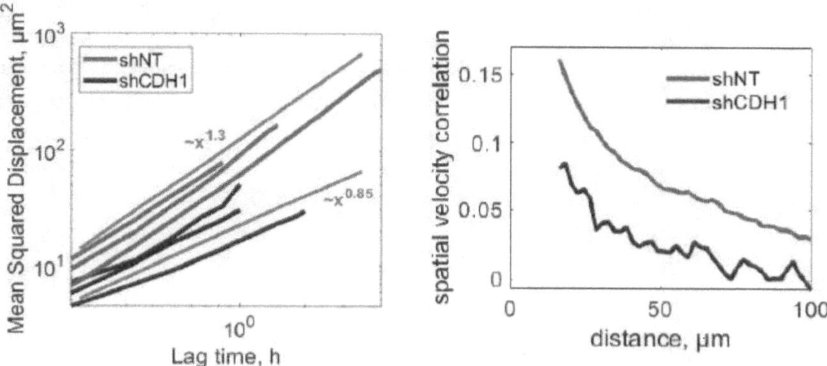

Figure 4.22: Analysis of *in vivo* tracks of cell nuclei. The mean squared displacement of the nuclei motion is plotted in the left graph, while the spatial correlation of the velocity of this motion is shown on the right side. The correlations are estimated using Pearson correlations and smoothed with a Gaussian kernel. [33]

The critical difference between the motion of E-cadherin^{high} and E-cadherin^{low} cells are transferable to the *in vivo* mouse model. The left graph in figure 4.22 shows the mean squared displacement graphs of the tracked nuclei. The E-cadherin^{high} cells again have a superdiffusive exponent, signalling their tendency of persistent motion. The exponent of E-cadherin^{low} cells is again lower, and in this case indicates subdiffusive behaviour, caused by many cells being stuck. As said before, the low amount of data reduces the confidence slightly, but the fact that the difference stays consistent is a good sign. The right side displays the spatial velocity correlation of the tracked nuclei, which again shows the same trend as *in vitro*. The spatial velocity correlation of E-cadherin^{high} cells is significantly higher than those of E-cadherin^{low} cells, indicating a collective behaviour for E-cadherin^{high} cells and a individual behaviour for the cells with down regulated E-cadherin. The spatial velocity correlation here was just a correlation of the velocity in x and y dimension, because the distance between z-slices makes the z-velocity quite noisy. For the distance between cells, the three-dimensional distance was used.

An important point, connected to this data is that the group of Prof. Friedl did not find any significant differences in the ability of these cells to metastasise in mice [33]. Traditionally, a further progression in the EMT, with down regulated E-cadherin, would be thought to be favourable for metastasis and one can also imagine the ability of cells to individualize to be important to cross barriers in the body. On the other side, the ability to move collectively and persistent can be of advantage in circumstances, where there is enough space to move. It is therefore not clear which of these phenotypes is more dangerous, and it very well might depend on the specific tumour environment. One has to keep in mind that the starting point of the E-cadherin down regulation in these experiments, the 4T1 cancer cell line, is described as an invasive, metastasising cancer cell line, that still has epithelial characteristics [44]. This means that the cell line already has acquired certain characteristics beside cell individualisation and a full EMT, that allow for metastasis.

4.3 Cell rearrangements within epithelial monolayers

In the previous chapters it was shown that an unjamming transition is possible by a loss of adhesion, increased cell shapes and decreased cell number density as well as volume fraction of cells. This does not mean that any of those factors individually is necessary or sufficient to unjam the system, even though, for example, a strong enough loss of volume fraction is clearly sufficient. It also does not prove, which processes are necessary for epithelial cell jamming in the first place. For example, I observed that a strong decrease in cell adhesion can unjam the system in chapter 4.2.2, but I did not observe the reverse effect of an increased adhesion during the transition between fluid and arrested behaviour in an epithelial cell layer in chapter 4.1.3.

The fact, that I was able to track the cell nuclei automatically, instead of using particle image velocimetry, which is usually used to asses the dynamic state of cell layers, allows me to study the individual cell behaviour. This aims at the core of jammed behaviour: Individual cells should be caged by their neighbours. If this is true, the structural properties of the local environment have to exhibit a strong influence on the dynamic properties of the cells. The automated tracking allows me to tackle this question for the first time and to investigate the importance of different parameters. This might not unveil the cell biological reasons for the jamming transition, but strengthen the coarse grained framework used to describe the collective properties of tissues. The tracking data used in the following chapter is the same data of arresting epithelial-like MCF-10A layers that is used in chapter 4.1, allowing comparisons to the development of the dynamics in the system as a whole.

4.3.1 Influence of tissue structure on rearrangement dynamics

The most obvious way to measure the rearrangement dynamics in a tissue are T1-transitions, as they are the minimal topological transition required for cell rearrangements and therefore are often used in theory and simulations [227, 30, 228]. Sadly, as shown in chapter 4.1.2, T1 transitions of tessellations around nuclei are to noisy in experiments, as even small fluctuations of the nuclei positions and detections of nuclei centres can lead to apparent T1 transitions in the experimental setting. This leads me to mostly use the magnitude of nonaffine displacement D_{min}^2, that was already introduced on chapter 4.1.1, to characterise the rearrangement dynamics. The advantage of D_{min}^2 in comparison to many other characterizations of glassy motion, like χ^2, is that it can be defined for each cell individually. It records the relative displacement of the cell in question compared to the mean movement of close-by cells, which in my case are usually the cells in 100 µm radius, minimised over all possible affine transformations. This provides a lower bound of the local tissue rearrangement and is already used in the literature of glassy systems [222, 216, 217].

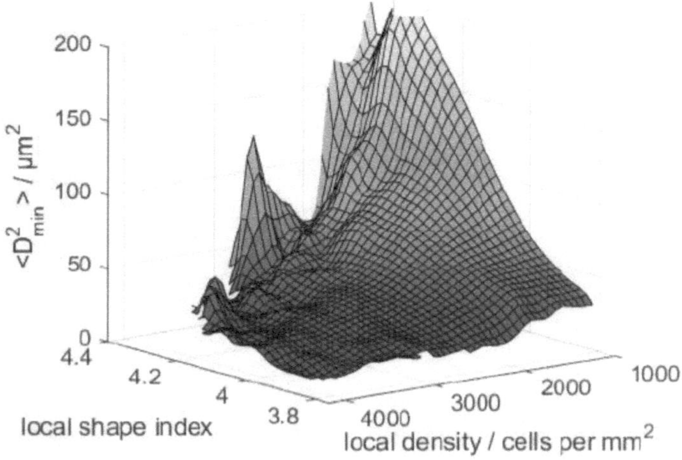

Figure 4.23:   The magnitude of nonaffine displacement D^2_{min} of cells in a confluent layer plotted over the mean shape index and cell number density of the cell and its neighbours. The individual data points are averaged with a two-dimensional Gaussian kernel.

The following graphs show relation of the local rearrangement dynamic to the structural properties of the local environment. The data set is restricted to the confluent period, because this is the time period, where cell jamming becomes possible and only the Voronoi-tessellation gives a good approximation of cell features. Figure 4.23 depicts the mean nonaffine displacement of cells within 2 hours, averaged over the mean local cell shape index and the local cell number density, whereby 'local' stands for the cell and its neighbours. The structural properties are recorded at the start of the time period that is used to asses the rearrangement behaviour. In this sense, the local structure predicts the rearrangement dynamics. The magnitudes of nonaffine displacements are ordered according to the local shape index and cell number density of the cell environment and averaged with a Gaussian kernel. Both of these structural properties have a large influence on the rearrangement dynamics of the cells, which already underlines the influence of the local environment and points to caging effects. As expected, these caging effects are characterised by a dynamical slow-down at high cell densities and round cell shapes. The lowest magnitudes of nonaffine displacement is found for cells that have an environment of densely packed and round cells, but cells that have either an extremely packed or round environment also tend to exhibit low amounts of rearrangements. Consequently, the highest values of nonaffine displacements were found for cells in sparse and elongated environments.

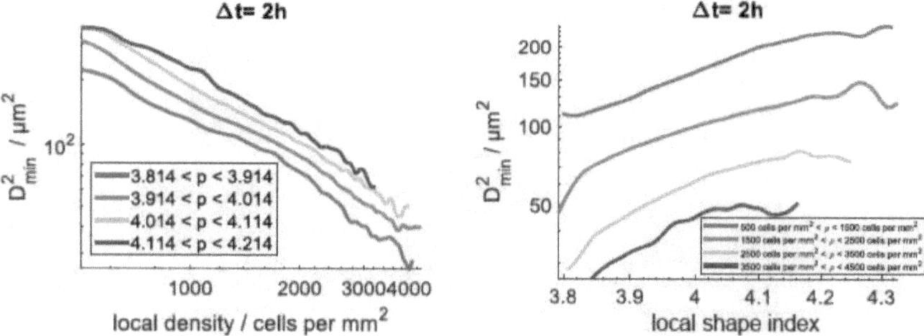

Figure 4.24: Sections of the previous graph that show the relation of the nonaffine displacement to the local cell number density ρ and local cell shape index p with the other parameter binned. The data again includes the confluent periods of the experiment and is smoothed with a Gaussian kernel.

This behaviour is also reproduced in figure 4.24, depicting the dependency of the rearrangement dynamics on the local shape index and cell number density, with the curves binned for the other parameter. Again, the word local describes the mean value of the cell and its neighbours and the structural parameters are recorded at the beginning of the two hour time period that is used to estimate the rearrangement behaviour. The data is smoothed with a Gaussian kernel and plotted in log-log plots.

The rearrangement intensity is reduced for increasing local cell number density and decreasing local shape parameter. Both of these plots show a roughly linear appearing relation with the magnitude of nonaffine displacement D^2_{min} and the respective local structural parameter in the log-log plot. This is normally a sign of a power law relationship, but the measured range of parameters is obviously to small to make such claims. The nonaffine displacement spreads nicely for the individual bins in the manner expected and shown in the respective other graph. Especially the different bins of the environment depending on their mean shape index appear to be very similar and only sequentially shifted up or down. This will be further discussed in the next chapter by rescaling the graphs on one curve. The graphs of the different bins of the local cell number density are sequentially shifted up and down too but also have slightly different slopes. It is apparent that the local cell number density has a higher spread of its bins in the right plot of figure 4.24 and covers a wider range of D^2_{min} in the left graph. This documents the importance of the cell number density for the ability of epithelial cells to rearrange.

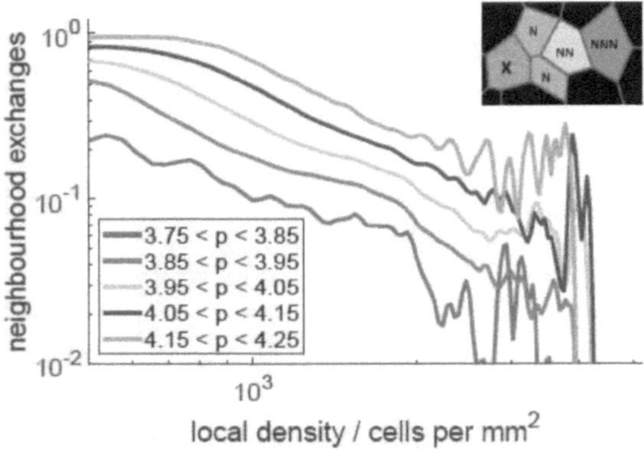

Figure 4.25: The neighbourhood exchanges, a direct measure of the ability of the cell layers to rearrange, plotted over the local cell number density and binned for the local shape index. A neighbourhood exchange happens when a cell receives a new neighbour that did not share a neighbour with the cell in question at the start of the time period of 4 hours. The topological distance that a cell has to traverse is indicated in the insert. Again, the term 'local' describes the mean value of the cell and its neighbours and the structural parameters are recorded at the beginning of the time period of four hours used to estimate the rearrangement dynamics via the neighbourhood exchanges. The data is smoothed with a Gaussian kernel and plotted in log-log plots.

Figure 4.25 depicts the analogy of the left graph of figure 4.24 in the metric of neighbourhood exchanges, which was already introduced in chapter 4.1.2 and is a direct, experimentally robust measure of topological rearrangements within tissues. For each cell, it records the amount of new neighbours that did not share a neighbour with the cell in question at the start of a certain time period, in this case four hours. This requires at least three T1-transitions. The main point I already made in chapter 4.1.2, but want to repeat here, is that the behaviour of this topological measure resembles the behaviour of the measure of the magnitude of nonaffine displacement D^2_{min}. From my point of view, this is a nice validation of the meaningfulness of both measures. The plot of the neighbourhood exchanges becomes very noisy in the regime of very high densities. The reason for this difference to the magnitude of nonaffine displacement D^2_{min} is that the amount of neighbourhood exchanges for individual cells can only be a natural number. The measure therefore needs a high amount of data points to accurately describe a nearly arrested system, where these neighbourhood exchanges still occur but only very infrequently. This, together with the fact that it is already an established measure, is the reason why I prefer to use the magnitude of nonaffine displacement D^2_{min} for the rearrangement analysis.

4.3.2   Rescaling of the influence of local cell shapes

As a reminder, on the left side of figure 4.26 the previously shown figure 4.24 is plotted again. It depicts the dependence of the magnitude of nonaffine displacement D^2_{min} on the local cell number density with bins for the local cell shape index. I already discussed previously that the different bins for the local cell shape appear to be similar and are sequentially shifted.

This sequential shifting, and the fact that the shifted distance is roughly constant for this range of shape parameters, suggests the possibility of the rescaling of the rearrangement. This is done in the right graph of figure 4.26 by the difference of cell shape index of the environment to a critical cell shape index $p^* \approx 3.81$ potentiated by an exponent that was found by trial. The overlap of the rescaled curves is not absolutely perfect, but looks quite good for a biological system. Already the fact that this rescaling is possible is very interesting since it resembles the scaling near a critical order parameter of a phase transition. In contrast to other properties of systems that are rescalable near phase transitions, the magnitude of nonaffine displacement does not diverge near the predicted critical point, but could potentially be inversely related to parameters that do diverge, like the cluster size of moving cells. In situations where cells can only move in enormous clusters the movement in a local environment will statistically appear affine. If I was using a topological variable like T1-transitions or

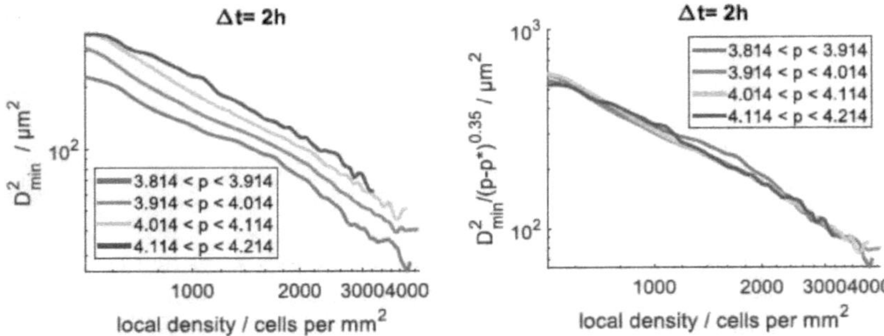

Figure 4.26: The left graph shows the relation of the magnitude of nonaffine displacement to the local cell number density binned for local cell shape. These structural properties are recorded at the start of the two hour time period used to estimate the rearrangement dynamics with D^2_{min}. The data includes the confluent periods of the experiments and is smoothed with a Gaussian kernel. The right graph shows the same data and plots the the magnitude of nonaffine displacement rescaled with the distance of the particular shape index to the critical shape index of $p^* \approx 3.81$ [31].

the neighbourhood exchanges discussed above, one could argue that the variable might implicitly depend on the order and shape of the neighbourhood, but this is not the case. The magnitude of nonaffine displacement is calculated purely by velocities and is therefore a priori not dependent on the shape of the cell neighbourhood. This means that this rescaling describes an effect that the structure of the cell environment has on the ability of the cell to rearrange. In other words, this rescaling is connected strongly to the caging effect that the local environment has on jammed cells. While the rescaling effect is quite robust, the rescaling exponent is dependent on the exact data set and time period used to estimate the magnitude of nonaffine displacement D^2_{min}, as I will discuss later.

Figure 4.27 shows results of simulations that Prof. Bi Dapeng performed in order to reproduce the rescaling behaviour shown above. The simulation is based on his published work of the SPV model, that I have summarised in the background chapter 2.2. In this coarse grained model, the simulated cells do not develop heterogeneities in the local cell number density and Prof. Bi did not observe strong correlations of the nonaffine displacement D^2_{min} to the local cell size. However, he did observe a family of curves similar to figure 4.26, by plotting the dependency of the local nonaffine

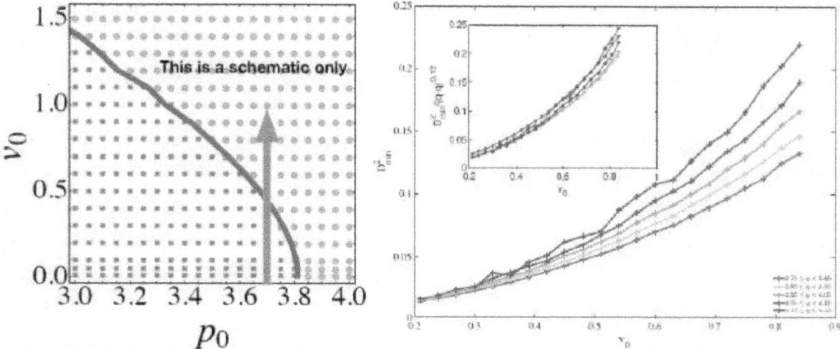

Figure 4.27: The left graph is a schematic based on the state diagram of the SPV model published in [32], illustrating the generation of the family of curves shown in the right picture. The right graph shows the magnitude of nonaffine displacement D^2_{min} in units of cell sizes depending on the internal velocity and binned for the local shape indexes. The insert shows the rescaling of these curves reproducing the experimental results of figure 4.26. The cell shape index is denoted as q in the right graph. The figure was produced by Prof. Bi Dapeng with the aim to reproduce my results in with his model.

displacement on the model parameter of the intrinsic motility v_0 binned with the local cell shape index. This family of curves can be rescaled with the same procedure as the experimental data shown before.

These results suggest two conclusions about the experimental data. First of all, the rescaling of the local rearrangement dynamics by the mean cell shapes of the environment can be reproduced by the model of shape-dependent cell jamming. This is a strong evidence that this model captures at least parts of the reality well. Density-driven jamming models might also be able to reproduce these findings, but a priori there is no reason that I am aware of that they definitely will. This means that these results could progress the ongoing discussion about the fundamental driving force of cellular jamming. The other conclusion suggested by this data, is that an increasing number density within an already confluent cell layer might have a glassy slow-down effect on the intrinsic cell velocity. This statement is motivated by the parallel between the experimentally observed correlation between the rescaling dynamic with the local cell number density and *in silico* use of the intrinsic motility to replace the local number density. It is quite reasonable from a cell biological perspective with different possible explanations in mind. The first one is the restructuring of the cytoskeleton from a motion oriented stress fibre containing state to an actin cortex dominated state, exemplified in chapter 4.1.3 and in recently published work like Saraswathibhatla et al. [190]. Other possible contributing factors can be cell-cell signalling cascades and the long known effect of contact inhibition of locomotion (CIL) [241]. This is the first analysis of experimental data I have seen, that can disentangle the effects cell shape and cell number density on cellular jamming. Of course, the data presented is not a final proof of the described interplay of shape and density effects, but provides a good first description and starting point for further experimental and theoretical work.

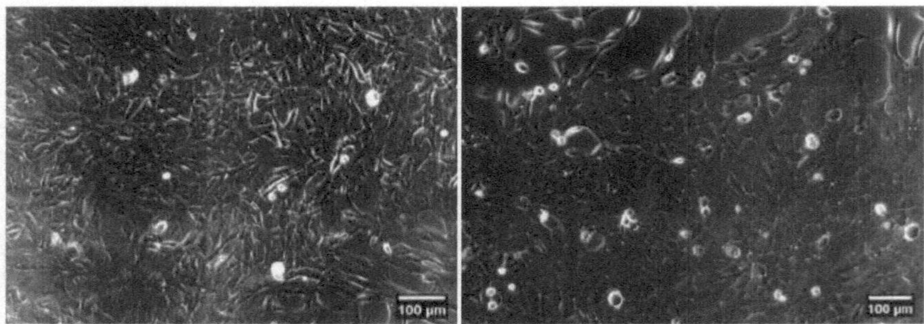

Figure 4.28:   Phase contrast images of MCF-10A cell layers, that are part of the presented tracking analysis. The left image shows section of a confluent epithelial layer, that has not yet developed a typical epithelial structure. The right image shows section of a non-confluent layer that has already, for the most part, developed a typical epithelial structure.

The next point I want to tackle is the rescaling exponent and how it depends on the time used to estimate the rearrangement behaviour. Before I do so, I have to provide a little more detail about the behaviour of the epithelial-like MCF-10A cell layers, since it turns out that the rescaling exponent strongly depends on the exact constrictions on the underlying data. When I recorded the times, where the experiments became confluent, I noticed that there consistently is a time point where the layer develops an epithelial-like structure. This can be before, after or simultaneous to the layer becoming confluent, depending on the initial density of the experiment. Example images of a confluent layer, that has not yet a typical epithelial as well as a non-confluent layer that already developed an epithelial structure are shown in figure 4.28. There are very small cell free regions in the left image, which I classified as confluent, but those are very unstable and open and close fast. Please excuse the medium quality of the phase contrast images, which were not the focus of these experiments designed to track the cells by their fluorescent nuclei.

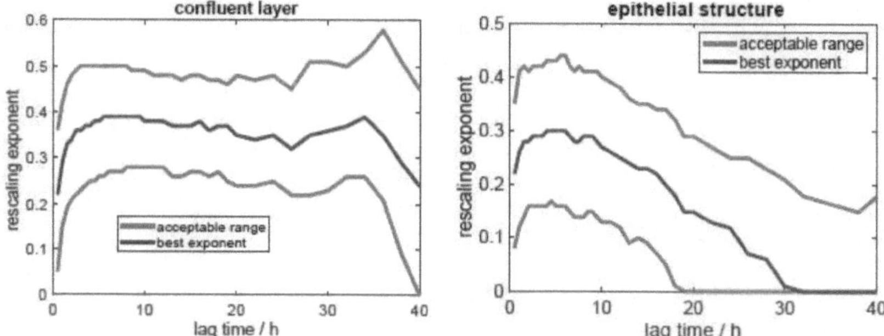

Figure 4.29: The rescaling exponents to rescale the magnitude of nonaffine displacement D^2_{min} shown in figure 4.27 depending on the time period used to estimate D^2_{min}. In the left graph only data point in confluent cell layers where used. In the right graph only data points in cells layers showing a typical epithelial structure where used. The acceptable range depicts the minimal and maximal rescaling exponents that cause a median standard deviation of the rescaled graphs lower than 10 percent of the median value of the graphs at the respective points. The best exponent the exponent causes the minimal median normalised standard deviation of the rescaled curves.

Figure 4.29 shows the dependency of the rescaling exponents introduced in figure 4.27 depending on the time period used to estimate the rearrangement dynamics with D^2_{min}. For this purpose, different rescaling exponents were tried and the standard deviation of the rescaled curves at each point was recorded and normalised with the mean value of the curves at this point. The median value of the thus normalised standard deviation were recorded and used to estimate the quality of the rescaling exponents. The red lines in figure 4.29 depict an acceptable range of the rescaling exponent as a kind of error bar, which shows the minimal and maximal values where the median normalised standard deviation is below 0.1. For the best exponent, which is produced by the minimum of the median normalised standard deviation, a slight smoothing was done before taking the minimum, since the values near it are quite close and fluctuate.

The initial expectation for studying the relation of rescaling exponents was a decrease in the rescaling exponent over time, until it reaches zero, and the family of curves shown in figure 4.26. The reason for this expectation, is that the mean cell shape index of the environment is recorded at the start of the time period used to estimate the respective magnitude of nonaffine displacement. When the rearrangement dynamics is studied long enough, the initial conditions should be forgotten over time. In this view, the decrease of the rescaling exponent and the time when it reaches zero could give information about the caging time of the cells in the system.

The initial point of surprise is that the rescaling exponents stay very high even for long lag times, describing a very long memory of the respective initial conditions in the system. Furthermore, it is apparent in figure 4.29 that this expected decrease is only occurring, when only data points were used where the layer was exhibiting an epithelial-like structure. In contrast, the best rescaling exponent of confluent data points does not decrease much for increasing lag times. One can explain this by postulating that the epithelial-like structure is an indicator for the jamming transition. This would mean that one averages over the fluid and jammed phase when one incorporates all confluent data points. Since the fluid phase can access parts of the phase space that are not accessible later and has significantly different dynamics, one does not average these away with longer lag times and the memory of them is still relevant. This interpretation suggests that the transition to the epithelial looking structure of the cell layer is very relevant to the transition to a jammed state, even more so than the time point, where the layer becomes confluent. The interesting observation in this context is, that both of these time points are usually not far away from each other and there is still a strong difference in the behaviour of the rescaling exponent visible. This suggest a quite sudden transition between the states, that is not as visible in the other analysis of the system, for example in figure4.5 and figure 4.9. The other sudden change, that was observed during the evolution of the epithelial-like MCF-10A layer was a fast reduction of the cortical contractility of the cell near the time of confluence. This suggests a connection between both of these effects, that would be consistent with recent publications connecting the cell contractility with state of mobility [190]. However, at this point it is not a clear statement but a direction for further research.

In a similar vein, I plotted the decrease in the rescaling exponents for data sets that start 5, 10 and 15 hours after the layer starts to look epithelial-like, in order to check how consistent the behaviour is. The overall behavior in figure 4.30 looks very similar with a plateau of the rescaling exponent for low lag times and a decrease to zero for higher lag times. However, the drop to a rescaling exponent of zero is shifted slightly

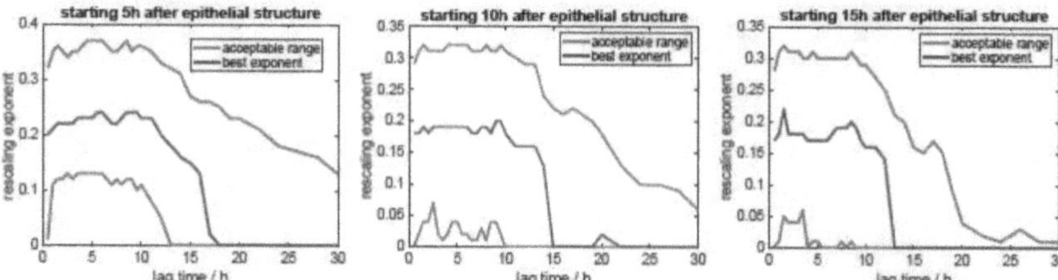

Figure 4.30: The behaviour of the rescaling exponents regarding the magnitude of nonaffine displacement D^2_{min} is shown in figure 4.27 depending on the time period used to estimate D^2_{min}. The data set is oriented to the time point, where the layer develops the epithelial-like structure, but a sequentially longer and longer time period after the development of an epithelial-like structure is discarded.

from 17h to 13h for increasingly selective data sets, that should be more and more arrested, since the motility of the cell in the layer is only reduced over time. This behaviour is at odds with a view of the decrease of the rescaling exponent to zero as an estimation of the caging time, since the caging time should only increase when the layer gets more arrested. I interpret this behaviour, similar to the argumentation before, as a decrease in the accessibility of fluid behaviour over time, which therefore restricts the accessibility of important parts of the phase space further, resulting in a decreasing memory effect. The caging time can not be extracted from this data set and is presumably also variable during the transition into the jammed system. I believe that one could use this procedure to estimate the caging of a fully quasi-stable jammed layer using a long observation time.

4.3.3 Predicting tissue rearrangements

As already described, the figures above indicated statistical predictions of the rearrangement of cells from their local environment, since the structural properties are recorded just at the start of the time period in which dynamic properties are measured. This leads to the attempt to use other tools of modern data analysis in order to predict rearrangement dynamics of the cell layer by its structure. In this case I refer to machine learning algorithms. I revived help in the use of the machine learning from Dimitrij Tschodu.

I recorded 46 different structural properties of the closer and wider environment for individual cells at each time point, in order to correlate them with the rearrangement dynamics of the cell. The kind of structural properties are the cell shape, cell number density and their variability. Another estimation of the cell number density used here, because it is window-size independent, is the distance to the 20th nearest neighbours. Another included parameter is the experiment time. The sequentially larger environments are the cell in question, the mean of the cell and its neighbours, the mean of all cells within a radius of $50\,\mu m$, $100\,\mu m$ and $200\,\mu m$ and lastly the mean value of the imaged section of the layer.

The algorithm tries to predict which cells are in the group of the 20 percent fastest rearranging cells only using structural features, as was done previously in a similar approach to investigate the effect of the environment in glasses, that inspired me [216, 217]. I employed Random Forests algorithms, since they can robustly handle outliers and the problem of collinearity in input parameters, using an ensemble of decision trees making a prediction by a majority vote [218]. I utilised the permutation feature importance, where the data of each feature is randomly permuted and a prediction is then made and compared to the unshuffled prediction accuracy [225]. More of the procedure is described in chapter 3.0.3.

As a minor point, I want to state that I compared different dynamic measures, and the magnitude of nonaffine displacements was the measure that was best predictable by the structural properties of the cell environment and layer. This is an indication of the robustness of the measure.

The data used for this machine learning analysis contains only cells in confluent cell layers. Initial tests included non-confluent data, which made the prediction of fastest rearranging cells very easy for the algorithm, which basically detected the non-confluent cells by using the global and local cell number density. The reader may be wondering, why I did not use the time point where the layer develops an epithelial-like structure, which is discussed in the previous chapter to specify the data of interest for the machine learning algorithm. Frankly, this is just a factor of timing. I performed the analysis presented here before getting clues about the possible importance of this time point and right now I just do not have any possibility to redo the machine learning analysis, for reasons of time constraints. It would be interesting to compare the outcomes for these slightly different data sets. Getting back to what I actually did: I sorted out cells, that had a cell division or cell death in the immediate neighbourhood, detected by the beginning or end of a track, because these are known to disturb the local environment increasing the local dynamic [211, 212] and I was interested in the 'ground state' of the tissue structures influence on its dynamics. This overestimates the amount of cell death and division, since it includes tracking errors, but there is enough data left and I do not see a potential bias, that is included by excluding cells with close by tracking errors.

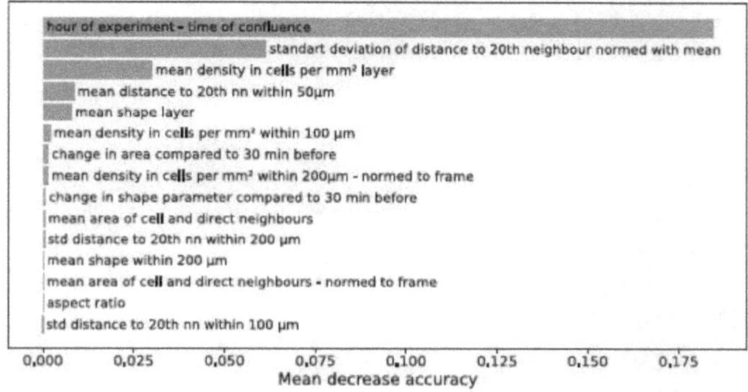

Figure 4.31: Feature importance for predicting rearranging cells with a high magnitude of nonaffine displacement using structural features of the layer via a of a random forest machine learning algorithm, which had an accuracy of 0.76. The data shown is the mean decrease in accuracy of the machine learning algorithm, when randomizing the data of the respective property.

The machine learning analysis, containing only confluent data, achieved an accuracy of 76 percent in deciding which cells are among the 20 percent of cells with the highest magnitude of non-affine displacement D^2_{min}, whereby the test ensemble consists to 50 percent of those fast moving cells and to 50 percent of slower moving cells. Only structural parameter and the experiment time are used for this decision. This is a very promising accuracy for an active and diverse biological system, as it is quite close to even the 80% accuracy achieved for glasses of simulated predictively similar particles [216]. The best predictor of dynamic behaviour, was not a typical structural parameter, but the experiment time, standardised with the time point at which the layer became confluent. The probable reason for this high importance is that there are still relatively fluid regions in the layer when it just gets confluent. At later times, even when cells are able to rearrange once within their neighbourhood, they will not get much further because of the high density. This means, that in this data set, which describes the transition from fluid to solid behaviour, most of the 20% of fastest cells exist early on in the confluent layer. Besides that, there might be biological ageing effects that occur during this period that slow down the rearrangements over time. Different possibilities are listed in chapter 4.1.3 and the only change that I observed was the restructuring of the cytoskeleton from a stress fiber containing one to a cortex dominated actin network. Another factor is the ageing of the medium, which certainly plays a small role, but is not the dominant factor in the ageing of the layer as one can reassure oneself by considering figure 4.9. Overall, this is also the explanation, why the accuracy of the prediction is this high for this data set.

The second most important structural feature, according to the machine learning analysis, is the standard deviation of the distance to the 20th nearest neighbour, which was used as a window-size independent estimator of local number density fluctuation of the layer. This is explained by the tendency of the epithelial cell layers to smooth out cell number density fluctuations by migrating into less dense regions. Thereby, they introduce rearrangements in this region, but also homogenise the density distribution of the layer reducing this driver of cell movement.

Other important parameters according to the machine learning analysis are the mean cell number density of the layer, the mean number density in the local region of $50\,\mu m$ and the mean cell shape of the layer. It is interesting that most of these parameters describe the structural properties of larger regions and not of small environments. A likely reason is, that there are still fluid regions in the data set, that the machine learning algorithm identifies. Jamming as a whole is a collective process and therefore the importance of the state parameters averaged over large regions makes sense. Both, the mean cell number density of the layer, as well as the mean shape index of the layer are highly correlated with the experiment time, but were also correlated with the rearrangement dynamic discussed in the previous chapters. The importance of the other parameters is so low, that they are not reliable at all.

Since there is such a pronounced layer effect of the experiment time in the data, I was interested whether the current structure of a cellular environment can predict the magnitude of rearrangement of this cell compared to the other cells at the same time. To prepare the data set for this analysis, I mapped the magnitude of nonaffine

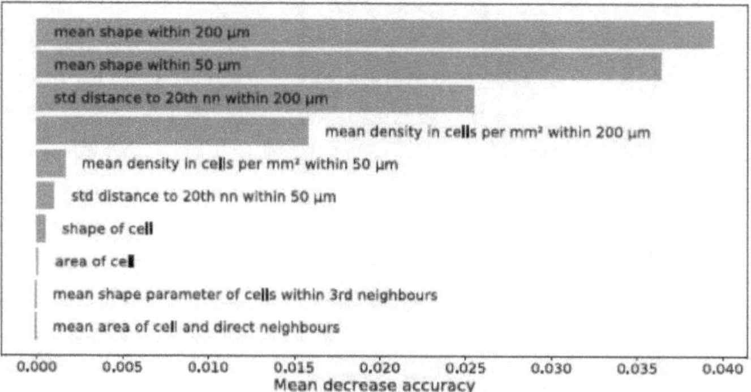

Figure 4.32: Feature importance for predicting the 20% fastest moving cells in each frame, according to the time normalised magnitude of nonaffine displacement, using structural features of the layer via a random forest, machine learning algorithm, which had an accuracy of 0.57. The data shown is the mean decrease in accuracy of the predictions, when randomizing the data of the respective property.

displacement D^2_{min} for each individual frame to a Gaussian distribution, whereby the ordering of the rearrangement magnitudes did not change.

The accuracy of the random forest algorithm is reduced drastically to 0.57 for this data set. This is not to surprising, since the task is drastically harder, but it renders the word predicting a little boastful, as 0.57 is not that much better than chance. This low prediction power also makes the different feature importances harder to interpret, because it is not clear whether they are only good at predicting a certain sub type of fastly rearranging cells or the system or data is just too noisy.

Since the rearrangement magnitudes are compared frame by frame, it is clear that parameters averaged over the whole frame do not play a role. Three of the four important parameters are still averaged over a large region, which underlines the collective nature of cell jamming, that was a little neglected by the discussion in this chapter, but is of course well known [21, 193, 242]. The two most important parameters for this prediction, where the mean cell shape index within 200 µm and 50 µm. This might be a small hint, that the local rearrangement is indeed shape dependent when one can discard temporal changes, but I have to state again, that the reliability of this evidence is rather small due to the low prediction accuracies. The third most important parameter is the standard deviation of the distance to the 20th nearest neighbour of each cell within 200 µm, which was used as a window-size independent measure of cell number density fluctuations. As discussed previously, it is logical that regions with high cell number density fluctuations show high rearrangements. The forth most important parameter, and the last parameter that shows a significant importance at all, is the mean cell number density within 200 µm. It is less important than the cell number density fluctuations similar to the predictions that were not normalised in time, but in this case the mean cell number density is well below the influence of the corresponding cell shape index.

4.4 Unjamming within densely packed three-dimensional tissues

While there are many different scenarios where jamming and unjamming is relevant for two-dimensional systems, like the epithelial surface of tissues and the unjamming occurring in asthma [26, 164], cancer progression is not one of them. Carcinoma, which are focus of this work, develop out of two-dimensional epithelial into three-dimensional tumour masses early in their development before they metastasise [104]. The malignant type of this carcinoma is called adenocarcinoma. Readers of chapter 4.2 already know that cancer cells can, under the right conditions, retain some epithelial traits and still be invasive. It is well known, that cancer is a very heterogeneous disease and challenging to treat, because it develops because of random mutations in cells of the body [243, 244]. This motivates the study of the physical framework that underlies the modes of mobility that tumours can use in order to develop criteria that can predict the kind of metastasis that these tumours are able to achieve. This requires an understanding of jamming and unjamming in densely packed three-dimensional tissues. The publication that resulted from this work is currently under review.

Spheroids of cancer cell lines are an ideal controllable system to study the dynamical behaviour of tissues in three dimensions. I will start by describing the possible differences in the dynamic behaviour of cell spheroids, connect these with the tissue structure and later describe how transferable these results are with respect to real tumour tissue. In contrast to the system in chapter 4.2, the spheroids are not influenced by boundary conditions, as they are self-contained on a non-adhesive surface. I received help from Steffen Grosser, Linda Oswald and Frédéric Renner with the experiments presented here.

4.4.1 Tissue dynamics in 3D spheroids

For this study, epithelial-like MCF-10A cells and mesenchymal-like MDA-MB-436 cells were used. These breast cancer cell lines that are often used to represent the transition between epithelial and mesenchymal properties [45, 245, 246, 170]. A visualisation of the spheroids used is given in figure 4.33a by confocal cross sections through the equatorial plain of exemplary fluorescently stained spheroids. The nuclei were stained with SiR-DNA and are coloured red, while the actin was stained with Alexa Fluor™

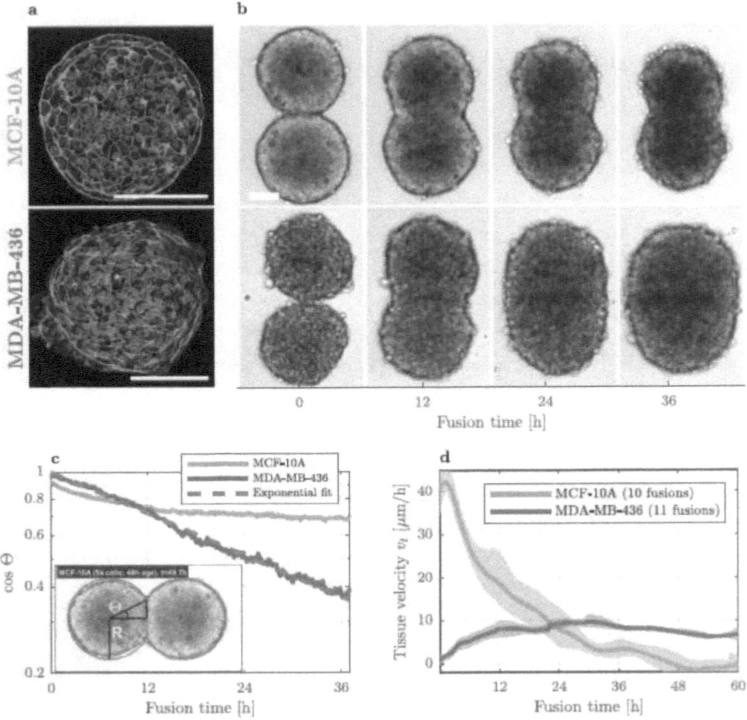

Figure 4.33: **a)** Confocal images of the equatorial plane of fluorescently labeled epithelial-like MCF-10A spheroids and mesenchymal-like MDA-MB-436. The actin signal is green and the nucleus is displayed in red. The scale bar represents $100\,\mu\mathrm{m}$. The global contrast is adjusted. **b)** A time series of phase contrast images of spheroid fusion experiments. The fusion of MCF-10 spheroids in the upper line arrests after roughly 12 hours. The scale bar represents $100\,\mu\mathrm{m}$. **c)** Classification of the fusion behaviour on exemplary spheroid fusions using the angle Θ between the spheroid center, center of the fusion neck and the edge of the fusion neck, visualised in the insert. The cosine of the angle Θ changes between one for two touching spheroids and zero for completely fused spheroids. **d)** Averages over 10 and 11 fusion experiments of the tissue velocity, that can be estimated by the change in Θ over time. The coloured areas are estimations of the confidence interval by bootstrapping.

488 Phalloidin and is displayed as a green signal. The scale bar represents $100\,\mu m$. The structure of the spheroids will be discussed later in more detail within chapter 4.4.2, but a few statements can be deduced already from the exemplary images. In contrast to some of the spheroids of chapter 4.2, the spheroids shown here do not contain any visible holes and are therefore at least close to volume fraction one. The spheroids consisting of epithelial-like MCF-10A cells appear visually more orderly than the spheroids containing mesenchymal-like MDA-MB-436.

The use of cell spheroids allows me to deploy one of the simplest macrorheological experiments possible: The fusion of two cell spheroids of the same type. Figure 4.33b shows a phase contrast time series of an exemplary fusion experiment for both of these cell types. The different behaviour is already apparent in the raw images: The fusion of MDA-MB-436 spheroids continues steadily over time, while the two epithelial-like MCF-10A spheroids arrest in a state of partial coalescence in the shape of a dumbbell. In order to quantify the fusion process, an edge detection was used an two overlapping circles were fitted onto the found edge, as indicated by the orange line in the insert of figure 4.33c. This insert also shows the construction of the fusion angle Θ, which forms the angle between the line that connects both spheroid centres and the line between a spheroid center and the edge of the fusion neck. This cosine of the angle evolves from one for two touching spheroids to zero after a completed fusion during the process. This analysis was motivated by Flenner et al. [14], who estimated the fusion of fluid cell spheroids of the same size with:

$$\cos\Theta = \exp(-t/\tau_{fusion}) \tag{4.2}$$

Thereby, the fusion time-scale τ_{fusion} can be connected with the spheroid properties with [14]

$$\tau_{fusion} = 2 \cdot R_S \cdot v_t = 2 \cdot R_S \cdot \eta \cdot \sigma \tag{4.3}$$

whereby R_S is the spheroid radius, v_t is the tissue velocity, η is the effective viscosity and σ is the surface tension. The predicted exponential for fluid-like spheroids fits very well to the observed behaviour of the fusion of MDA-MB-436 spheroids, as shown in figure 4.33c. On the other hand, the epithelial-like MCF-10A spheroids do not at all show an exponential behaviour in the decrease of $\cos\Theta$. This observation gets accentuated by considering the change of the tissue velocity, which can be estimated by the slope of the of the cosine of Θ:

$$v_t(t) = -2 \cdot R_S \cdot \frac{d}{dt}(ln \cos \Theta) \qquad (4.4)$$

The development of the $\cos\Theta$ is averaged slightly over time to reduce the influence of noise in the experiment and edge detection. The time development of the tissue velocity is plotted in figure 4.33d as an average over 10 and 11 fusion experiments for MCF-10A and MDA-MB-436 spheroids respectively. After some initial time to get started, the tissue velocity connected to the mesenchymal-like MDA-MB-436 spheroids is roughly constant at about $9\,\mu m\,h^{-1}$. On the other hand, the tissue velocity of epithelial-like MCF-10A cells starts very high at about $40\,\mu m\,h^{-1}$, but is steadily reduced to zero within 48 hours. This vanishing of the tissue velocity is a strong indicator for a jammed behaviour of the spheroid, or at least the core of the spheroid. In theory, it could also be explained by an increase in the viscosity of the system to nearly infinity, which one could call a glass transition, or the vanishing of the surface tension over time. An indicator of the surface tension are the cells on the surface, which are very elongated for MCF-10A spheroids. This indicates a high surface tension for this spheroid type and does not change much with time, as one can insure oneself by considering the figures 4.37 and 4.38. The high surface tension is consistent with results of epithelial layers in 2 dimensions [247], and provides an early explanation for the initial high fusion velocity of the MCF-10A spheroids.

In order to further investigate this behaviour and solidify the previous claims, cell spheroids were observed live. These experiments require smaller spheroids, to allow the imaging of the inner part of the spheroids with a Spinning Disk Laser Scanning Microscope (LSM), which is of confocal nature. It is not enough to just image a region of the same distance below the surface, because the spheroid can not be stopped from rotating slightly, which can be fixed in the post processing by a 3D image registration for small spheroids, but would move the region of interest in a large spheroid out of the observed part. The nuclei of these smaller spheroids were stained with SiR-DNA and observed with a 5 minute interval. The spheroids used in this experiments were one day old. Considering any possible ageing effects, they correspond to the behaviour within the first 24 h of the spheroids in the fusion experiment.

The results of these live observation experiments are summarised in figure 4.34. Part a of this figure visualises the spheroids used by a 3D rendering of one of the frames of the time series, using a FijI [208] plugin called 3D viewer. It is hard to visualise

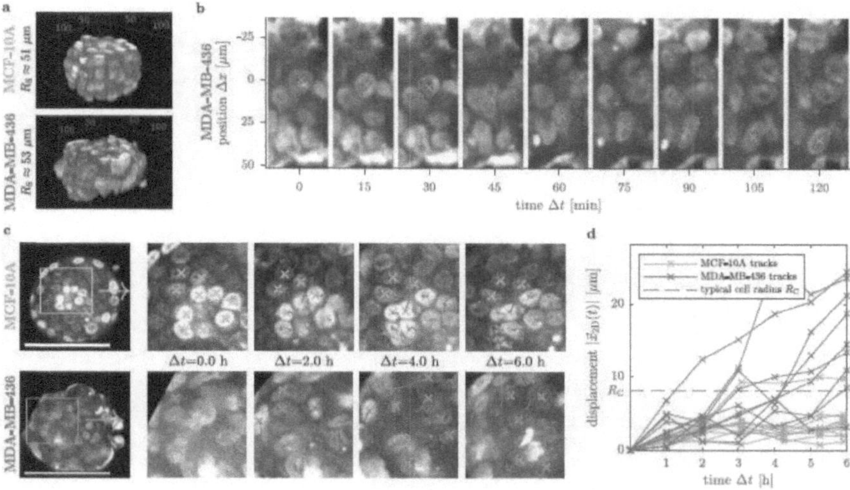

Figure 4.34: **a)** Three-dimensional rendering of one frame of a three-dimensional time series of spheroids with fluorescently labelled nuclei (SiR-DNA), that are displayed in grey. The spheroids contain about 200 cells and were imaged every 5 minutes. **b)** An exemplary time series of a cell within a MDA-MB-436 spheroid, that is able to move through different environments. The cell nuclei is coloured red for clarity and moves through 7 z-stacks corresponding to roughly 24 µm and a total relative distance of about 40 µm within 120 minutes. **c)** Manually tracked cell nuclei of MCF-10A and MDA-MB-436 spheroids, with crosses as nuclei indication and orange track indications **d)** Displacements of the tracked nuclei shown in c.

the impression of motion in these four-dimensional data sets. The MCF-10A spheroids appear quite static on the inside, while the MDA-MB-436 spheroids exhibit much more relative nuclei motion. An example of an outstandingly moving cell is featured in the time series of figure 4.34b. The nucleus of this cell is highlighted in red and marked with a blue cross. The fluorescence signal of the other nuclei is shown in gray. The first and last sections of the time series are 7 z-stacks or roughly 24 µm apart. The cell moved about 40 µm respective to its surrounding within 2 hours in a dense three-dimensional environment. Even though this is just a drastic example, this movement is a strong confirmation that MDA-MB-436 cells are able to rearrange themselves in their spheroids. It is apparent that the cell nucleus elongates during the cell movement and occasionally elongates extremely, when it has to squeeze through a very dense environment. While it is just an individual counter example, the motion of the cell in minute 45 is a strong argument against the notion that a dense cellular environment alone is sufficient to jam tissues, as the cell is able to move a tiny gap and even narrower gaps in all directions are hardly imaginable. This is in accordance with experiments of very narrow artificial tunnels, that seldom stop the crossing of cells completely [248]. Those provide a firm environment that allows cells to generate strong forces and the experiment presented here is one of the first ones to demonstrate the rearrangement of cells in realistic extremely dense cellular environments.

The aim of this experiment was to generate an automatic tracking of nuclei, but the experimental conditions turned out to be too challenging using confocal Spinning Disk LSM. The fluorescence quality was very variable in time and between cells, possibly because of the rotations of the spheroid that are managed by an image registration. In addition, MDA-MB-436 cells that change places with others, or squeeze between other nuclei, come very close to them, which obstructs an automatic cell tracking. With an automatic cell tracking being unreliable, a selection of 10 cells for each cell type in an exemplary and well stained region were tracked by hand. Most of these tracks are displayed in part c of figure 4.34. The tracked nuclei are marked with crosses(green or blue) and the tracks are indicated with orange lines. The background shows the fluorescent nuclei in grey and also exhibits some freshly proliferated cells, which are a good sign for the health of the sample. The tracks of MDA-MB-436 cells show movement, that lets them exchange places and neighbours within the 6h time period. In contrast, the MCF-10A cells for the most part only show very slight motion and out of the 10 cells only one moved enough to change neighbours and non of them did move enough to switch places with another cell.

Part d of figure 4.34 shows the time displacements of the tracked nuclei compared to the position in the initial frame. MCF-10A tracks are plotted in green, MDA-MB-436 tracks are plotted in blue and a typical cell radius of $R_c = 8\,\mu m$, known from cell segmentations presented later, is indicated as a dashed orange line. Nearly all of the epithelial-like MCF-10A cells move substantially less than the typical cell radius R_c, while all of the mesenchymal-like MDA-MB-436 cells moved more than the typical cell radius R_c in the period of 6 hours.

This information provides an indication about the state of the spheroids, even with the sparse amount of data. Consider the Lindemann criterion [249], that connects the particle movement to the state of the system by introducing a threshold fraction δ_L of the inter-particle distance that signifies a fluidisation of the system within a particular time scale, if the particle movement in this time scale exceeds this fraction of the inter-particle distance. For atomic and molecular systems the threshold fraction typically lies in the range of $0.05 < \delta_L < 0.22$ [249, 250, 251, 252]. For this system some additional considerations have to be made: The cells and cell nuclei are elongated and the latter can move inside the cells without forcing cell movement. In order to give a rough estimation of the amount of movement that a nuclei is capable of inside a cell, I will preempt results from the next chapter dedicated to the analysis of cell shapes. Typical cell shapes of the segmented cells have an aspect ratio between 1.5 and 2, denoting that the nucleus has about a factor of $\sqrt{2}$ more space in the elongated direction than one would expect for completely round cells. A thresholding of the nuclei signal of spheroids gives an estimation of the nuclei volume of roughly 30%-40% of the cell volume. This provides an estimation of the nucleus radius of $R_N \approx 0.35^{1/3} \cdot R_C \approx 0.7 R_C$. This combines into the conservative estimation of the additional room for non-fluidizing movement of the nucleus of: $\delta_{intracell} \approx \sqrt{2} * (2 * (R_C - R_N)) \approx 0.85 R_C$. Accounting for these possible intracellular fluctuations, an estimation of the fluidisation threshold of $\delta_L \approx 0.5 \widehat{=} R_C$ seems useful for this system.

The displacement curves in figure 4.34d show tracks of MDA-MB-436 cells that all cross this estimation of the Lindemann criterion and most of them do it drastically. Only the one MCF-10A track, that managed to change some of its neighbours during the 6 h time period crosses this threshold and most of the other displacement curves do not even reach half of this value. Thus, the Lindemann criterion suggests a fluid behaviour for the MDA-MB-436 spheroids and a solid behaviour for MCF-10A spheroids, which is consistent with the macro-rheological spheroid fusion experiment. The exact value of the estimated threshold factor δ_L is not of prime importance for this statement. The predicted macroscopic state would not change by doubling or halving the approximated additional intracellular wiggling room for the nucleus.

The fusion of the MCF-10A cells slows-down over time and completely arrests after 2 days. The tracking of the cells in the core of the spheroids suggests, that it already behaves solid-like within the first day. This suggests that the shells of the spheroids are more fluid than the inside and can rearrange until the fusion would require the core of the spheroids to rearrange themselves. Another possibility is that the surface tension overcomes the yield-stress of the jammed spheroids at the beginning but is less and less able to do so over time, because the rearrangements that take place reduce the exerted stress. I will discuss this further after the structure of the spheroids is classified.

It is interesting, that the movement of the MCF-10A cells within the spheroid did not seem completely frozen. The prime example is the one nucleus, that was able to change neighbours, which stayed at his initial place for 2 hours, moved rather quickly and stayed at his next position for the rest of the observation time of 3 hours. This occasional sudden movement does seem more typical for a jammed system, inducing caging effects, than for glassy motion, where the core description is that the motion is frozen out and the relaxation times diverge.

4.4.2 Structural properties of 3D spheroids

The previous chapter demonstrates fluid-like cell behaviour for MDA-MB-436 spheroids and solid-like cell behaviour for MCF-10A spheroids. This section is dedicated to connect these different dynamic behaviours to the structural properties of the spheroids.

The first important statement is that the spheroids do not contain any appreciable amounts of cell free spaces, in contrast to the spheroids of the E-cadherin down regulated phenotype in chapter 4.2. This is demonstrated in figure 4.35, that shows a MDA-MB-436 spheroid labelled with CellTracker Green suspended in a dextran solution labelled in orange. The same approach has been used in other systems to detect cell free regions [53]. Here, no open, orange labelled spaces are visible at cell boundaries, certifying that the volume fraction of the MDA-MB-436 spheroids is close to 1. The dextran check was done for MDA-MB-436 spheroids because they were questioned to be volume filling, because their fluid-like behaviour is typically connected to a non-confluent structure, like for the system in chapter 4.2.

One of the parts of the actin cytoskeleton is the actin cortex, that is situated under the cell membrane at the edge of the cell. Images of fluorescently stained actin can therefore be used to estimate the boundaries of cells and with them the cell shapes and sizes. Figure 4.36 shows an illustration of such a cell shape analysis. The equatorial plains of example spheroids is shown in the upper row, with the signal of fluorescently stained actin in green, fluorescently stained nuclei in blue and indications of the boundaries between segmented cells in red. These images are part of a three-dimensional representation of the spheroids via confocal stacks. In order to achieve a good image quality, necessary for a cell segmentation, the spheroids were fixed before staining and cleared afterwards (see protocol section A.5). The automated cell shape segmentation relies

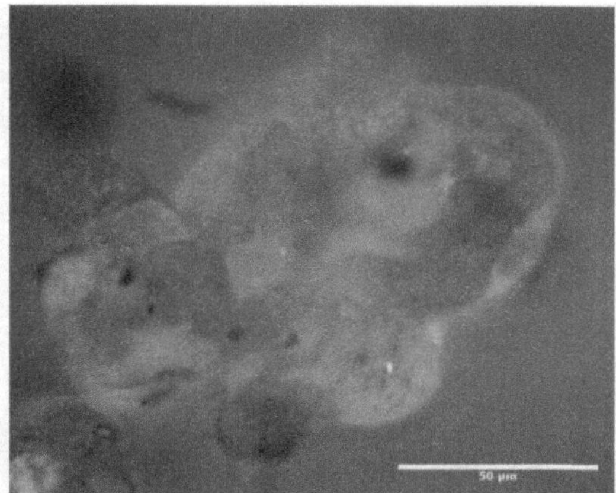

Figure 4.35: Confocal slice through the middle of a small MDA-MB-436 spheroid labelled with CellTracker Green in a dextran solution labelled in orange. The scale bar depicts 50 µm.

on an identification of the cell positions by the nuclei and an elaborate combination of water shedding of boundary information constructed out of the actin and nuclei fluorescence signal which is followed by smoothing and error corrections described in the methods chapter 3.0.2. The segmentation is one of the first developed segmentations that work fully in three dimensions. As one can see by inspecting the example images in the upper row of figure 4.36, the segmentation works well for most cell outlines, but is not error free. This is acceptable, because the statements derived from it are using average values and large ensembles and can at least qualitatively be double checked by the visual impression of the system. I would not put too much stock in the exact reported values, but they are probably close to the real value and the relative differences between the ensembles are reliable, as one can convince oneself by considering the error analysis in the method section 3.0.2

The first impression generated by the fluorescently stained equatorial slices is that there seem to be no, or only very tiny, cell-free regions within both of these spheroid types. There is typically only one maximum of the fluorescence signal in the line of the actin signal between two cells, which means that the actin cortices of both cells are closer together than the optical resolution of approximately 250 nm. This is a confirmation of the control experiment shown in figure 4.35, and different to many

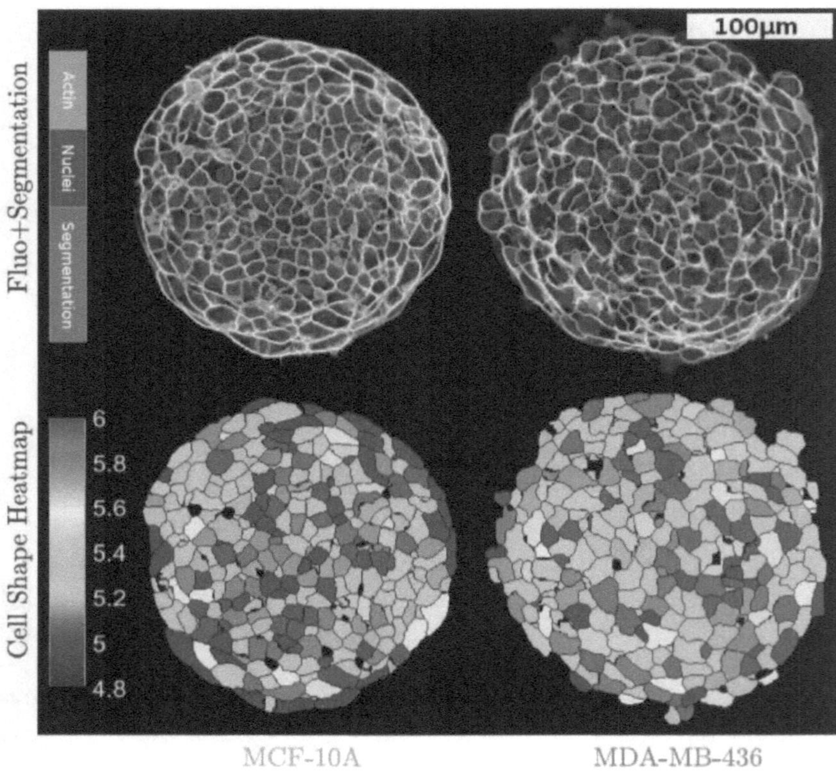

Figure 4.36: The equatorial plains of MCF-10A(left) and MDA-MB-436(right) spheroids are displayed in the upper row. These are part of 3D stacks of confocal fluorescence images. The actin signal is shown in green, the nucleus signal is shown in blue and the boarders of my automatic cell segmentation are shown in red. Red areas signal the boundary of cells in z-direction. In the bottom row, a heatmap visualises the 3D cell shape of the segmented cell shapes. The plotted value is the shape index of the ellipsoid with the same second moment as the segmented shape.

other studied systems, like the one in chapter 4.2 or in Mongera et al. [53]. Therefore the observed fluid behaviour of the MDA-MB-436 spheroids occurs at volume fraction one and a transition between the solid state of MCF-10A spheroids and the fluid state of MDA-MB-436 spheroids is possible without a change in the volume fraction of the system.

The segmented fluorescent images evoke a visual impression of a more ordered state for the solid-like MCF-10A spheroids and a comparatively disordered state for the fluid-like MDA-MB-436 spheroids. One reason for this intuitive classification is the straightness of most MCF-10A cell boundaries, compared to boundaries seen in MDA-MB-436 spheroids that are often more wiggly. On the level of the image processing, this is caused by more pronounced and straighter actin cotex structures in MCF-10A cells compared to MDA-MB-436 cells. This difference in the actin structure is already a clue to a possible cell biological origin of the change in the motile state, as similar effects are reported in chapter 4.1.3 and the literature [190]. This visual impression of differences in the actin cortex structure is in accordance with recent measurements of the cortical contractility of both cell types [206].

Another reason for the impression of higher orders in the MCF-10A spheroids is visualised more clearly in the bottom row of figure 4.36. This row shows a heatmap of the 3D cell shape index of the cells that are part of this equatorial plane. The exact measure used is the three dimensional cell shape index S_e of the ellipsoid with the same second moments as the segmented cell. Thereby the cell shape index is defined as the ratio of surface area divided by volume to the power of two-thirds, making the parameter dimensionless. The ellipsoid with the same second moments than the segmented cell shape is interjected to reduce the influence of the outermost surface of the segmented cells, which is prone to noise and the exact algorithm used for the cell segmentation. The bottom row of figure 4.36 shows that the core of MCF-10A spheroids have comparably round cells, while their surface show very elongated cells that are arranged preferably parallel to the surfaces. The MDA-MB-436 spheroids have no apparent structure and the constituting cells appear more elongated than the inner cells of MCF-10A spheroids.

A quantification of these observations is shown in figure 4.37. The data is divided in MCF-10A and MDA-MB-436 spheroids with age of one and two days or two and three days after seeding, respectively. The reason is that the MDA-MB-436 cells need more time to form the initial spheroids. For the cell shape index, the upper graph in figure 4.37 verifies the statements indicated above, that the MCF-10A cells are rounder in the core region than MDA-MB-436, but more elongated at the surface. The surface elongation was already hinted at in the previous chapter as an indication of surface tension. It is remarkable that the high surface elongation of cells in the MCF-10A spheroids does not decrease over time, which is an indication that the surface tension does not decrease considerably, which refutes one alternative explanation of the arrest in spheroid fusion discussed in the previous chapter.

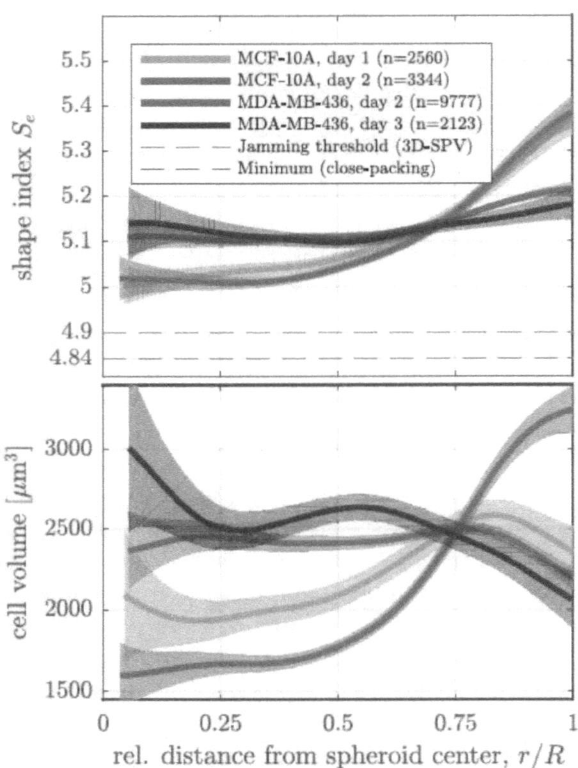

Figure 4.37: Moving averages of the mean cell properties depending of the position of the cell relative to the spheroid center. The shape index S_e is the three-dimensional cell shape index of the ellipsoid with the same second moments as the segmented cell. Multiple spheroids are averaged and the coloured areas depict the confidence interval corresponding to p=0.05.

The round cell shapes in the inside regions of the MCF-10A spheroids are in general agreement with the concept of a shape-dependent cell jamming transition, but the numerical value of the measured cell shape indices are higher than predicted in simulations [46]. The value of 4.9 indicated as the jamming threshold of the 3D SPV-model in the figure 4.37 is not the value of the shape index of 3D Voronoi cells within the publication of Merkel and Manning [46], but those of the corresponding ellipsoids with the same second moment than the Voronoi cell, in order to be comparable with the experimental data. This shows again, that the cell shape is a very important parameter in the cell jamming transition, but also that the transition is not completely described by the SPV-model, which has to come at no surprise considering the massive simplification and coarse-graining of the model.

Interestingly, not only the cell shape index but also the cell volume is reduced in the core region of MCF-10A spheroids, compared to the surface region and MDA-MB-436 spheroids. This increase in the cell number density is even more pronounced in older spheroids, that also show a lower tissue velocity in fusion experiments. The graph in figure 4.33 can also be explained by other factors, such as a decrease in the importance of the shell region, that already fused. However, in fusion experiments started with older spheroids, the fusion was slower and arrested earlier. It is important to distinguish the increasing number density from other cases, that reported an increasing cell density in the sense of volume fraction accompanying a solidification, for example in three dimensional embryo tissue [53]. In this view, the MDA-MB-436 spheroids are already in the confluent, most dense state. Similarly, in topological views of rearrangements, the number density of the system can not even enter easily as a parameter. Nevertheless, it is logically clear that it can play a role, considering that the material presumably gets stiffer in a denser state and is harder to push during rearrangements.

The observed differences between the inside and surface structure of MCF-10A spheroids, in both number density and cell shape lends credence to the hypothesis, that they might have an arrested core and an outer layer, that is able to rearrange, at least under outside stress.

Figure 4.38 illustrates the properties of the cells during the fusion process. The original spheroids are still discernible in the stage, where the spheroids were fixed. This presumably would stay that way for MCF-10A spheroids, where the fusion arrests and not a priori for MDA-MB-436 spheroids. These spheroids share the main features of the individual spheroids: Round cell shapes in the cores of the MCF-10A spheroids, that do appear unchanged, higher cell shapes in MDA-MB-436 spheroids and extremely elongated cells on the surface of MCF-10A spheroids that are parallel to the surface. In

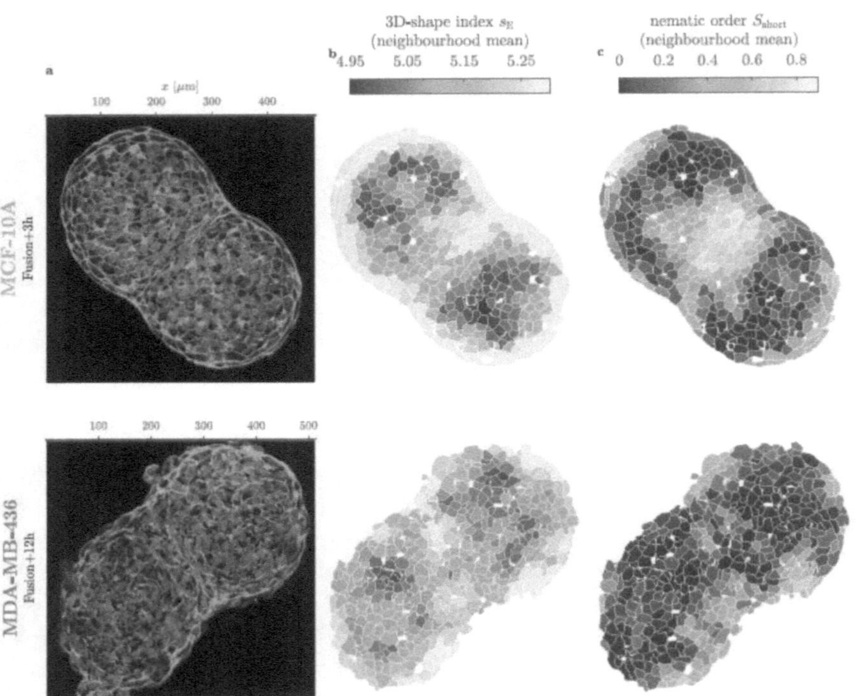

Figure 4.38: Cell shapes of spheroids fixed during the fusion process. The top row shows MCF-10A spheroids and the bottom row shows MDA-MB-436 spheroids. The first column, labelled **a**, shows the equatorial plane of the fluorescence images, with a red nucleus signal and a green actin signal. Column **b** shows a heatmap of the three dimensional cell shape index S_e of the ellipsoid with the same second moments, for the cells in the equatorial plane, locally averaged. Column **c** shows a median over the neighbourhood of a local nematic order parameter of the short axis of the cell. For each cell, its neighbours orientations are correlated with the orientation of the cell, to identify a local ordering. The white areas in column b and c do depict boarders between cells in z-direction and not cell free regions.

the middle between the original MCF-10A spheroids, the cells are still more elongated than in the core region of the original spheroids, but some of them are already rounder than cells in the shell region that build up this part initially. For MDA-MB-436 cells, the region between the initial spheroids does not have features distinguishing it strongly from the rest of the spheroids, although individual cells there might be very slightly more elongated.

The most striking feature visible in figure 4.38 is the alignment of MCF-10A cells in the boarder region between the initial spheroids. In order to quantify that, I use the local nematic order parameter of the short axis of the cells, defined as $S_{short} = \frac{1}{2}(3\cos^2(\alpha)-1)$ for all cells, whereby α is the angle between each cell and the mean orientation of its neighbours. Averaging this over the local neighbourhood provides a local nematic order parameter. The cells in the region between the initial spheroids of the MCF-10A cells are very oblate and the short axes are oriented with each other, as the high nematic order parameter in this region validates. The other axes are not aligned strongly, since the orientations of the longer axes of oblate cells is not robust. These results suggest, that at the beginning of the MCF-10A fusion many elongated, oblate cells are oriented in the same direction at the boarder between spheroids, which could conceivable cause a collective, directed motion, similar to wound healing and the system in chapter 4.2, where boundary conditions and cell alignment of cells with epithelial-like characteristics lead exactly to collective and directed motion. An interesting point here is that I observe an ordering of strongly oblate cells and not prolate, that is more usual for nematic-like ordering. The reason for this is clearly the initial ordering through surface tension, but after this system is initialised that way the usual steric arguments, first brought up by Onsager, still hold. The steric interactions are even harder to avoid for oblate particles, than for prolate ones.

There has been a variety of research about the influence of cell nuclei and their properties on the ability of cells to move, especially in the extracellular matrix [49, 50]. As the nucleus is the largest structure within cells and one of the stiffest, it is an obvious hypothesis that the nucleus is an important factor regarding tissue behaviour. The left part of figure 4.39 illustrates the main axis of a cell and its nucleus. Considering that image, it becomes evident, that nuclei in densely packed, elongated cells have to be elongated themselves, or they simply will not fit inside the cell. This is also apparent in the larger fluorescence images in figure 4.36 and 4.38. The right graph of figure 4.39 shows the distributions of the ellipsoid shape indices S_e, described before, for cell bodies and nuclei. The shape properties of the nuclei are calculated by spatially averaging the fluorescence intensity inside the segmented cells. The distributions are generated with 1 day old MCF-10A spheroids and 2 day old MDA-MB-436 spheroids, excluding the surface layer. It is evident that the general features of the distribution are shared

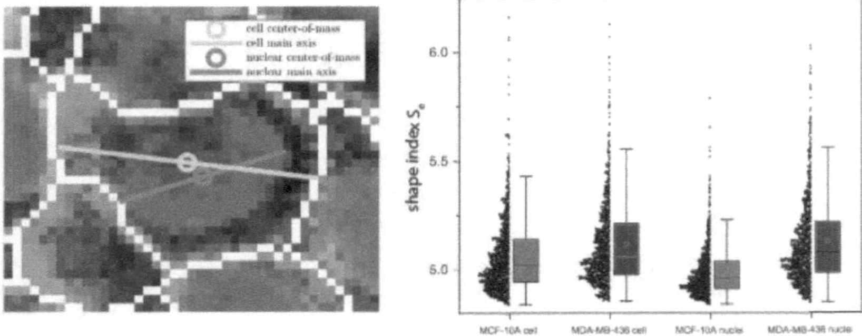

Figure 4.39: Quantification of nucleus elongation in spheroids. The left figure illustrates of the center of mass and the main axes of elongation of cell bodies and nuclei. The right graph depicts the distribution of shape indices of cell bodies and nuclei within one day old spheroids. The distributions are generated out of the cells in 1 day old MCF-10A spheroids and 2 day old MDA-MB-436 spheroids, excluding the surface layer. The black dots represent the individual cells and the box plots represent the quantiles, the middle line represents the median and the small square represents the mean of the distribution.

between the shape of the cell bodies and the shape of nuclei. For MDA-MB-436 cells, the distribution of the ellipsoid shape index S_e for nuclei is almost identical to the corresponding distribution for the cell body. For MCF-10A cells, the shape of the distribution is again very similar between to nuclei and cell bodies, but the nuclei are even rounder than the cell bodies.

Figure 4.40 shows that the correlation of cell and nucleus shape not only holds on an ensemble level, but also for individual cells. In this figure, the individual ellipsoid shape indices S_e of nuclei are plotted over the corresponding ellipsoid shape indices of the cell bodies. Similar to the ensemble values presented in figure 4.39, the nucleus shapes of MCF-10A cells are slightly rounder than the cell shapes, while both of these values are surprisingly similar for MDA-MB-436 spheroids. The high correlation between these two properties is recognisable by considering the narrow data cloud surrounding a linear appearing relation. This validates the logical and visual impression stated before, that nuclei in densely packed, elongated cells have to be elongated themselves, or they simply will not fit inside the cell. Thus, given that cells have to elongate to fluidise the

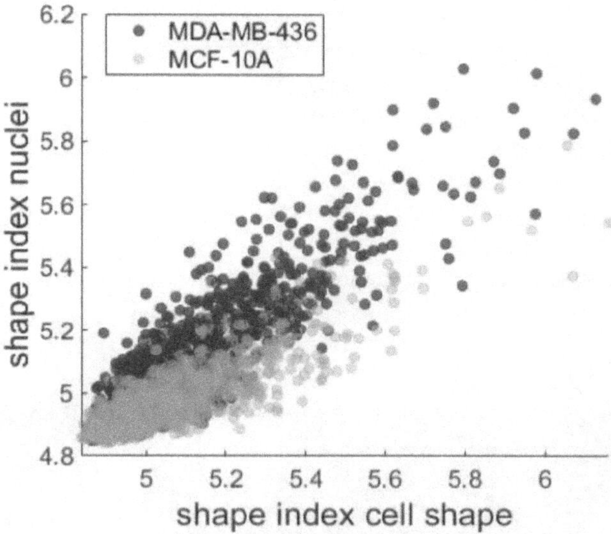

Figure 4.40: Individual nuclei shape indices plotted over the shape index of the corresponding cell body of exemplary MCF-10A and MDA-MB-436 spheroids.

system, as many observations in this thesis and elsewhere indicate, the deformability of the cell nucleus is presumably an important puzzle piece in the cell biology of the transformation between solid-like and fluid-like tissues. Another conclusion regarding this data is, that the shape of cell nuclei can be used as an indicator of the shape of densely packed cells, at least at an ensemble level. This is an important insight, since the nucleus shape is drastically easier to measure in fluorescent images and histological slides. It will also be used in the following chapter.

4.4.3   Comparison to tumour pieces

The previous two chapters demonstrated that densely packed three-dimensional spheroids can be in a solid-like or fluid-like state, accompanied by a high number density of cells and round cell and nucleus shape compared to a lower number density of cells and more elongated cells bodies and nuclei. All this research is motivated by its connection to cancer tissue and its behaviour, which will be discussed in this chapter. In order to accomplish this, I was part of a collaboration of my group with the University hospital Leipzig and I would like to thank Prof. Höckel, Prof. Aktas, Prof. Horn and their staff for access to primary tumour tissue of breast and cervix cancer. The collaboration includes many biophysical experiments and I will only present an excerpt of the project, that I was strongly involved in and that connects to the other work of this thesis.

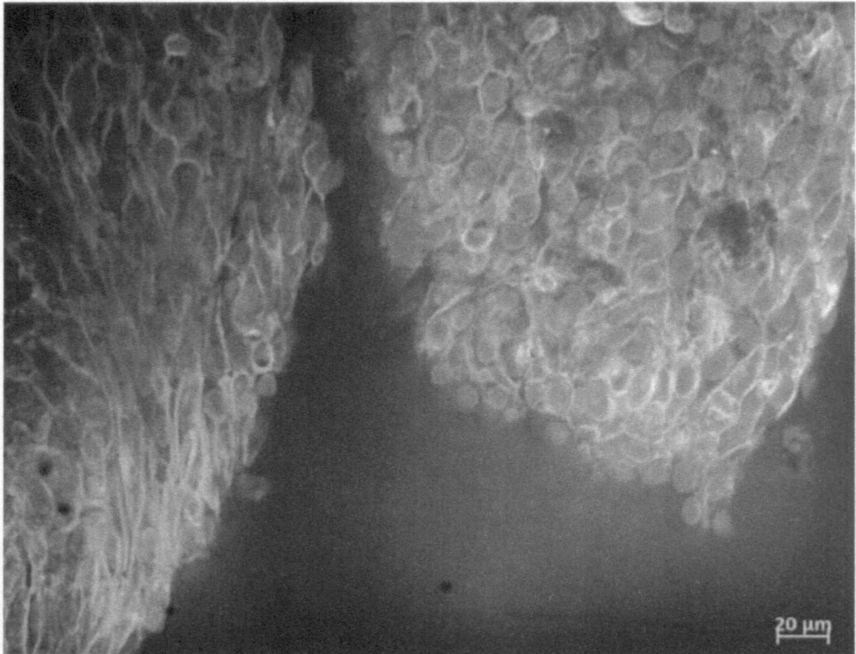

Figure 4.41: A piece of primary cervix tumour tissue with actin stained in green and nuclei stained in red.

Figure 4.41 shows one z-stack of a three-dimensional fluorescence image of a fixed piece of cervix tumour, where actin is stained in green and nuclei are stained in red. It is apparent that many of the statements about the structure of the cell spheroids also apply to this tumour piece. Large regions of the tumour are densely packed, without any cell free spaces. This means that the properties of densely packed spheroids studied above are very much relevant for real tumour tissue. Furthermore, there are regions with very elongated and partially aligned cells visible, as well as regions with drastically rounder cells, that are accompanied with a higher number density. This means that the results from the previous chapter would predigt a fluid-like behaviour in one of these regions (in the left part of the image) and a solid-like behaviour in the other region. It is also noteworthy that also in this system elongated cells contain elongated nuclei and rounder cells contain rounder nuclei.

In order to investigate the prediction, motivated by figure 4.41, that tumours can contain fluid and solid-like regions at the same time and that those are distinguished by their cell and nucleus shape, live tracking experiments, similar to those for the spheroids done in figure 4.34, were performed for small tissue pieces. An exemplary slide is shown in figure 4.42a. The orange tracks in this slide demonstrate nicely fluid-like and solid-like regions in the same tumour piece. The fluid-like characteristic of the region in the middle of the tumour piece can be recognised by the long tracks, that imply high cell velocities, and the uncoordinated route of the tracks signal a high relative cell motion and the ability of the cells in the tissue to rearrange. The bottom row of figure 4.42 shows a three-dimensional rendering of the spheroid shown in the upper image at a specific time point, as well as a confocal slice of a cleared and stained tissue piece. The main statement of these images is their resemblance of the corresponding images from cancer cell spheroids shown in figures 4.34a and 4.33a, which again is affirming the validity of these spheroids build up of cancer cell lines as a model system for my purpose.

The analysis presented here contains samples from 14 different patients. For most of them multiple small pieces resembeling those shown in figure 4.42 and 4.43. Not all of the tumour pieces contained mobile regions, but for all clinical stages of the patients, mobile regions were found insight the pieces. In other words, even early tumours contained fluid regions. Nearly all tumour pieces also contained solid regions. Figure 4.43 shows fluid and solid regions on another example tumour piece. The motile state of the regions were assessed by eye after studying the time series of 3D fluorescence images. Nuclei in these regions were tracked by the FijI plugin TrackMate [208, 207].

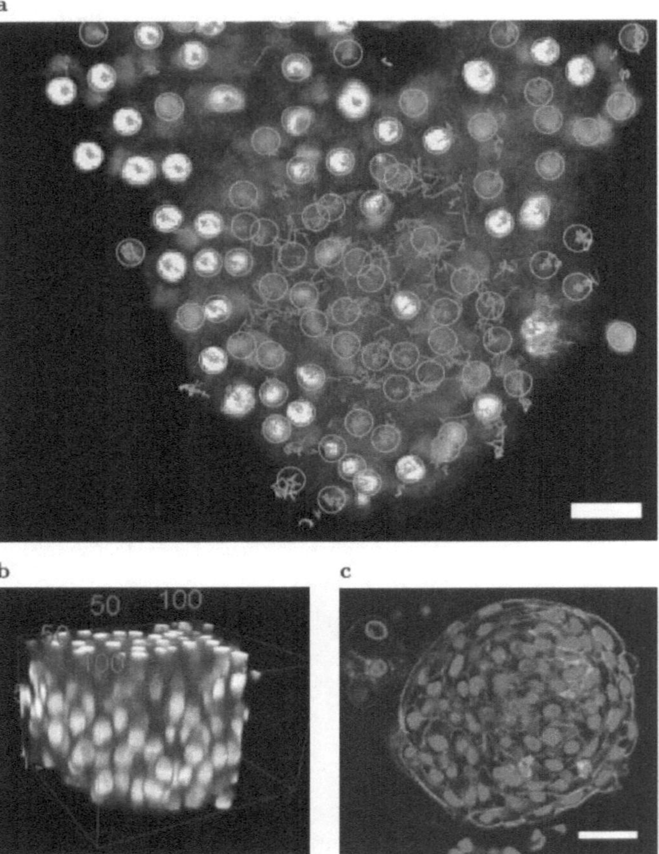

Figure 4.42:   **a** Small piece of primary tumour from a breast cancer patient, which was stained with vital SiR-DNA, observed for 12 hours and tracked using TrackMate [207]. A slice through the middle of the tumour piece is displayed, with the nucleus fluorescence in gray, detected nuclei marked with blue circles and indications of tracks marked in orange. The scale bar represents 20 μm. **b** 3D rendering of one time point of the live observation of the tumour piece shown in a using FijI [208]. **c** An exemplary slice of a fixed and cleared primary tumour piece, with actin stained in green and nuclei stained in red. The scale bar represents 50 μm.

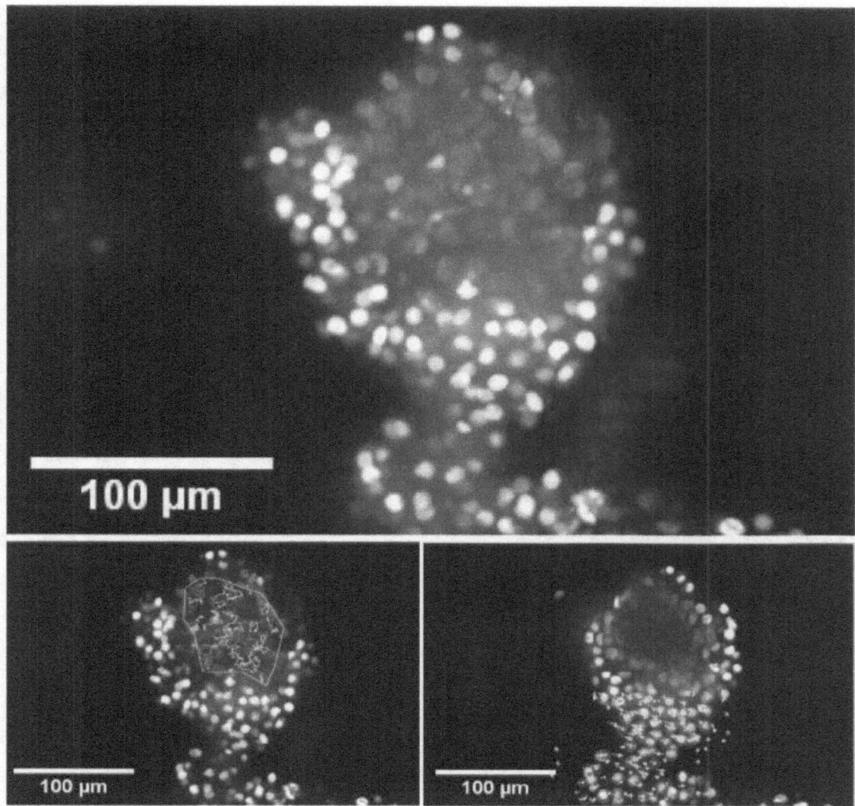

Figure 4.43: Another exemplary tumour piece. The upper image shows a close up a confocal plane in the middle of the piece. The bottom row indicates regions of fluidly moving (left) and arrested (right) cells. The regions were estimated and drawn by hand. The tracks shown were done using TrackMate [207].

Without going into detail, I want to state that the tracks validate the visual assessment of the motile states by having lower velocities and MSD's for the solid-like regions compared to uncoordinated, high velocity motion for the fluid-like regions. The fluorescence image without the overlaid tracks suggests a difference in the nuclei between the regions, that were identified as fluid and solid. The solid regions appear to have smaller and rounder nuclei, that seem to be usually also stained brighter with SiR-

DNA. I am not sure what the brighter stain is caused by. On the other hand, the differently elongated nuclei are an appealing point to focus on, since it corresponds well with the results of the spheroid analysis, where the fluid spheroids also consisted of more elongated nuclei, which were correlated with elongated cells.

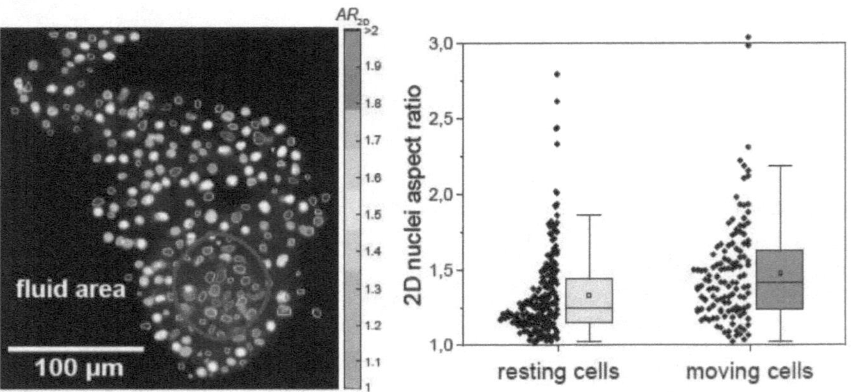

Figure 4.44: The left image shows fluorescently labelled nuclei in primary tumour pieces, which were segmented using the FijI plugin StarDist [208, 253]. The segmentations are visualised as lines around the segmented nuclei in the colour corresponding to the 2D aspect ratio of the nuclei. The right graph displays the 2D aspect ratio distributions of 130 moving nuclei and 229 resting nuclei out from primary breast and cervix carcinoma. The black dots represent the value of individual nuclei and the box plots represent the quartiles, the median with the line in the middle and the mean with the square.

In order to investigate the visual assessment, that the cell nuclei in the fluid regions are more elongated, the nuclei were connected to fluid and solid regions and segmented using the FIJI plugin StarDist which is a nuclei detection algorithm based on star-convex polygons [208, 253]. Since the amount of data is manageable, the quality of the segmentation was checked and falsely segmented nuclei were manually corrected. The left graph of figure 4.44 shows a visualisation of this segmentation by surrounding the fluorescence signal of the nuclei in the analysed confocal plane with lines surrounding the segmented nuclei. These lines are coloured corresponding to the two-dimensional aspect ratio of the segmented nuclei. This means, that not all nuclei that are elongated in three dimensions have to be detected as elongated here, because their longer axis can point in z-direction. On an ensemble level, a group of more elongated, and not perfectly aligned nuclei will still cause a higher distribution of two-dimensional aspect ratios [254].

The right graph in figure 4.44 shows the distributions of the two-dimensional aspect ratio of the segmented nuclei for the resting and moving cell regions. The distributions contain 130 moving cells with a median nuclei aspect ratio of 1.42 and 229 resting cells with a median nuclei aspect ratio of 1.26. The distributions of the aspect ratios are clearly different, as the upper quantile of resting cells barely reaches the aspect ratio of moving cells. The p-value of the corresponding Kolmogorov-Smirnov test is $p = 1.5 \cdot 10^{-6}$. This analysis validates in primary tumour tissue the conclusion from spheroids of cancer cell lines that fluid-like cell regions in densely-packed cell clusters are recognisable as regions with elongated nuclei in static images. As far as I know, this is the first time, that this connection is made and therefore the robustness of the finding in similar but different systems still has to be validated, but this is an exciting starting point for further research as it promises a hypothesis driven ansatz to quantify the properties of cancer samples in static images like histological slides. I will illuminate this idea more deeply within the following discussion section.

Chapter 5

Discussion

In the genetic and molecular framework, cancer is an extremely complex disease and very challenging to treat an diagnose [103, 6, 7, 8, 9]. However, these various molecular changes have to adjust the cellular properties in the physical world in order to achieve processes like metastasis. The framework of cellular jamming is an interesting candidate for a predictive model explaining how changing cellular properties lead to different motile states of cells and tissues [163]. This thesis proves that this framework indeed applies to tumours and develops it further by investigating the underlying causes of cell jamming. I will start this discussion section by shortly summarising the key achievements in each of these projects and continue by clarifying what the results of this thesis can contribute to the open questions in current research.

Since cell jamming is inherently a local effect, where cells are caged by their neighbours, it is an important step in the understanding of causes for cell jamming to measure the local rearrangements in systems close to jamming and quantify the properties that have an effect on them. This goes beyond any previous studies which only measured average properties of cellular systems [21, 27, 26, 178]. In the chapters 4.1 and 4.3 I present my study of tissue rearrangement dynamics in epithelial-like monolayers, with high temporal and spatial resolution. In these studies, I found no evidence that points to a first order transition between fluid-like motion and solid-like behaviour 4.1.1. The time development of the layer suggests a transition of higher order, which is consistent with theories that predict a linear increase of energy barriers starting at a critical cell shape [30]. The spatial resolution revealed that the rearrangement dynamics of cells is strongly dependent on the local cell number density and the mean cell shape of the cells neighbours. This justifies the terminology of local caging, which is often assumed throughout the literature (chapter 4.3.1). The rearrangement dynamics of cells can be rescaled by the mean cell shape of their local neighbourhood near the critical cell shape index predicted by theories of shape-dependent cell jamming (chapter 4.3.2) [30, 32]. This resembles critical scaling behaviour near a phase transition and is strong evidence that the cell shapes can function as the control parameter for cellular jamming in confluent disordered tissue. The parameter measuring the rearrangement dynamics does not diverge near the transition, but could potentially be proportional to the inverse of a divergent parameter. This is the first time that experimentally a scaling behaviour near a critical point is found between cell shapes and the state of motility in tissue.

In the development of cancer the behaviour of three-dimensional tissue is the important factor, which in contrast to two-dimensional sheets is hardly studied with respect to cellular jamming [25, 53, 188]. The investigation of densely packed cell spheroids in chapter 4.4 reveals both solid and fluid-like behaviour for different cell spheroids in bulk rheological measurements and cell movement. I was able to connect these states of tissue motility with the structure of the spheroids and showed that both round cell shapes and high cell number densities correlate with cell jamming in three dimensions. The mean cell shape index of the ellipsoid with the same second moments S_e corresponding to cells of solid-like MCF-10A spheroids in the core region is roughly 5.0 and thereby significantly lower than the corresponding cell shape index of fluid-like MDA-MB 436 spheroids with 5.1, but drastically higher than the predicted value for three-dimensional cell jamming at 4.9 [46] (see figure 4.37). The difference in cell number is currently not included in models of cell jamming, which either focus on the volume fraction of cells in the tissue or the effects of cell shapes [163]. Importantly, these spheroids are at volume fractions very close to 1, without any holes visible. Previously, the jamming and unjamming in 3D was experimentally connected only to changes in the volume fraction [53, 255] or linked to the intrinsic cell motility [188]. The cell shape and state of motility in the densely packed three-dimensional tissue was linked to the shape of the nuclei, which previously were only considered important in the context of cell movement in the extra cellular matrix [256, 49, 50]. This correlation between nucleus shape and motility in densely packed tissues is transferable to primary tumour pieces as shown in chapter 4.4.3, showing that round cell shape contribute to the energy barrier for cell rearrangements in tissues close to jamming.

Besides the investigation of the underlying causes of cell jamming in two and three dimensions, it is important which biological processes trigger the unjamming transition in cancer and how this relates to invasion and metastasis. Chapter 4.2, whose data was published in Nature Cell Biology [33], is concerned with the effect of down-regulation of E-cadherin on the state of motility in cancer spheroids in the presence of a collagen boundaries. E-cadherin down regulation is the prototypical process of the epithelial-mesenchymal transition (EMT), which is a central process connected to the development of carcinoma [231, 38, 232, 34]. The down regulation of E-cadherin in 4T1 cells, an invasive breast cancer cell line that still retains epithelial characteristics [43, 44], causes an increase in cell elongation, a decrease in number density and a loss of cohesion, which decreases the volume fraction of cells (chapter 4.2.1). This is accompanied by a switch from collective, persistent motion to individual, diffusive motion indicating a strong decrease in cell rearrangements (chapter 4.2.2). This change in the state of motility is consistent between *in vitro* experiments and experiments in mouse models. In contrast to the E-cadherin high original 4T1 cells, the E-cadherin down regulated cells could individually invade sparse collagen networks (2 mg/ml), but were also retained by denser 6 mg/ml collagen networks. Overall, this data is fascinating because it describes a fluidisation that occurs because of biological changes that also accompany cancer progression. Interestingly, experiments in mice did not find a significant difference between the ability of both cell types to metastasise.

Shortly summarising these results, I found critical scaling behaviour for the rearrangement dynamics of cells near the jamming transition, depending on the cell shape of the environment. This is the strongest evidence yet, that the cell shapes can function as the control parameter for cellular jamming. The cell number density also influences jammed behaviour, but its influence can be described as a slow down of the intrinsic velocity of cells, as I will discuss below. Thus, a high cell number density on its own would only increase the viscosity of the tissue and not solidify the system. This analysis of my data generates the prediction that there are no solid-like disordered tissues with elongated cell shapes. Furthermore, I showed that there is a jamming transition in confluent three-dimensional tissue that is connected to the cell shapes. I showed that there also exists a correlation between the motile state of a tissue and the shape of its nuclei. This is evidence that nucleus deformations, which need to be larger for round nuclei, contribute to the energy barrier for cell rearrangements in densely packed tissue. This new insight has clinical applications as it provides a physical explanation for the diagnostic marker of nuclei shapes in histological slides, indicating the possibility of developing a new predictive marker for the ability of cancer cells to metastasise. I also showed that E-cadherin down regulation, which is a typical step during cancer progression, causes an unjamming transition. There is a prominent loss of cohesion and a reduced volume fraction of cells in this particular unjamming transition, although it is also connected to elongated cell shapes. This shows another route of unjamming and proves that multiple conditions are required for jammed behaviour in tissues. These results show that an unjamming transition can occur during cancer progression and change the invasive behaviour of the cancer cells [33]. In order to develop a predictive framework using this process it is crucial to understand the mechanisms behind the cell jamming transition.

Cell jamming is caused by cell shape and density

Currently, there is a debate in the field whether cell jamming is a density-driven or shape-dependent phenomenon [21, 26, 31, 53, 47, 178]. Both in 2D and in 3D, the early publications that reported an arrest in cellular motion correlated it with increasing cell density and an increase in the volume fraction of the system [257, 53]. The volume fraction is also the parameter controlling granular jamming [258, 28], but the additional importance of the cell number density is only typical for cells, because of their high softness and deformability. This correlation is also visible in the data I present in the chapters 4.1 and 4.2 for monolayers and slices of spheroids, respectively. In some sense, this dependency of cell jamming on the volume fraction is the most basic dependency possible. It is logically clear that cells can not cage each other when their volume fraction is too low, because the caged cell would have too many degrees of freedom. A model of soft particles predicts a jamming transition around a volume fraction of 0.842 in two dimensions [28], and if an arrest of motility would occur at lower volume fractions it would be a strong indication that it is not caused by a jamming mechanism. If there exists an arrested, jammed state in cellular systems, it has to have a high enough volume fraction of cells in order for them to be able to sterically contain each other. The existence of fluid behaviour in confluent tissues, at volume fraction 1 or very close to it, proves that a high volume fraction is not a sufficient condition for jamming in cellular systems where the building blocks are self-driven and able to reshape themselves. The fluid behaviour of confluent systems has been shown for two-dimensional airway epithelium that undergoes changes related to asthma [26] and is, in 3D, the implicit basis of the classic differential adhesion hypothesis for cell sorting, which generally works for most types of tissue but specifically not when epithelial-like cells are involved [10, 12, 168, 170]. The MDA-MB-436 spheroids presented in chapter 4.4 are also examples of fluid-like three-dimensional tissues at volume fraction 1.

The idea of a shape-dependent cell jamming transition originates from coarse-grained Vertex-, Voronoi- and Potts-models of tissues, at first in two dimensions [30, 31, 32, 203]. For two-dimensional layers, correlations between the average cell shapes and the state of motility of the layers have already been shown experimentally [26, 179, 178]. Interestingly, it was not a priori clear, that the considerations leading to the shape-dependent jamming transition in theories of two-dimensional are transferable to three-dimensional tissues. The Hamiltonian used for the model of shape-dependent jamming has a quadratic term in the deviation of volume and surface area from the preferred cell properties, which can be understood as two constrains per cell. Compared to the cells degrees of freedom in three dimensions, which are 3 spatial degrees times the cell number plus one degree for an overall shear, the system is highly under-constrained [46]. The jamming transition only occurs in the three-dimensional model because degrees of freedom are frozen by residual stresses [46]. This uncertainty about the transferability of the mechanism of shape-dependent jamming to three dimension renders its experimental discovery in chapter 4.4 of high importance. As described above, I showed that densely packed spheroids can exhibit solid-like and fluid-like behaviour and proved that this difference in motility is correlated with cell shapes in three dimensions. These are the first results that show that the mechanism of shape-dependent jamming is relevant for tumours, as it was previously never observed for three-dimensional systems. This paves the way for further research connecting shapes of cancer cells with clinical outcomes.

Other data in this thesis, that provides new insights regarding shape-dependent jamming, is the study of rearrangement dynamics in epithelial-like cell layers. The rearrangement dynamics of individual cells measured by the magnitude of their non-affine displacement D^2_{min} can be rescaled by the mean cell shape of the cell and their neighbours near the critical cell shape $p* = 3.81$ predicted by Vertex models [30, 32]. This rescaling uses the distance to the theoretically predicted critical cell shape and therefore resembles critical scaling near a phase transition, which is the first time that more than a mere correlation between the cell shape and state of motility in tissues was shown. In contrast to other properties of systems that are rescalable near phase transitions, the magnitude of non-affine displacement does not diverge near the predicted critical point, but could potentially be inversely related to parameters that do diverge, like the cluster size of moving cells. In situations where cells can only move in enormous clusters the movement in a local environment will statistically appear affine. These are strong indications that the cell shape in confluent systems is the parameter determining the jamming transition and the effect of other parameters is only of modulating nature. This means that a disordered tissue with elongated cell shapes should never be in a jammed state and therefore allows to draw strong conclusions regarding the dynamics in tissues by observations of their structure. The qualifier of disordered tissue is inserted, because for example nematic structures could be special cases because their degrees of freedom are restricted in another way. Thus, the data presented in the chapters 4.3.1 and 4.3.2 contains very strong indications for a shape-dependent jamming transition in two dimensions, while the data in chapter 4.4 shows that these concepts are transferable to three-dimensional systems.

Besides this shape-dependence, there is also a strong correlation of the rearrangement ability of the tissues on their cell number density visible in the data throughout this thesis, which I will discuss in the following paragraphs. In the arrested MCF-10A spheroids, the core region consists of cells that are both rounder and have a higher number density. The same is true for non-targeted 4T1 cells compared to their E-cadherin down regulated brethren, especially on the inside of the spheroids. In this data it is not fully distinguishable which of these effects is the more important one, because non of these experiments were especially designed to do so. This problem occurs throughout the literature, where both cell number density and cell shape were found to correlate with the state of motility in tissues, often at the same time [21, 26, 164, 163, 185, 179, 53, 178]. The dynamic data with temporal and spatial resolution, presented in chapter 4.3 are able to provide some insights here. Similar to other studies, I also observe a strong correlation of the rearrangement dynamics with the cell number density, globally and locally. However, while it is possible to rescale the magnitude of nonaffine displacement D_{min}^2 of cells, measuring their rearrangement dynamics with the mean cell shape of cells in their neighbourhood, it is not possible to do that for the mean number density of cells. This provides strong evidence that the cell number density does not exhibit the critical scaling behaviour that the cell shape exhibits and is evidence that the main parameter of cell jamming is the cell shape. The influence of the number density of cells is therefore only a modulating factor, which is discussed in the next paragraph. Thereby, the curves of the magnitude of nonaffine displacement D_{min}^2 plotted over the local cell shape index for different local cell number densities in figure 4.24 become steeper for higher densities, which means that the influence of the cell shape becomes more pronounced for higher cell number densities. This also means that regions at very high density do not even reach states with very round cell shapes. They are jammed at higher cell shapes and can not rearrange further to reach lower cell shapes. This results mean that a dense environment amplifies the underlying shape-dependent jamming transition. The way in which this amplification likely happens is described in the next paragraph.

The influence of the cell number density on the rearrangement dynamics is hard to describe in geometric models, such as the vertex model that motivated the description of a shape-dependent jamming transition, as it is not an intrinsic variable in these scale-free models. My collaborator in this project, Prof. Bi Dapeng, reproduced the general behaviour of the interaction between rearrangement dynamics, cell shape and number density by replacing the number density with the intrinsic velocity with his SPV-model [32] (see figure 4.27). This means he can reproduce a rescaling of the rearrangement dynamics of simulated cells, by the distance of the mean cell shape of their environment to the critical shape parameter of his model, whereby the overall dependency is plotted over the intrinsic velocity of the cells in the system. This a strong indication that the effect of the cell number density on the rearrangement dynamics can be approximated by a slow-down of the intrinsic cell velocity similar to a decrease in temperature of glassy systems. This seems like a reasonable interpretation, since a loss of intrinsic cell velocity in confluent tissue is similar to a decrease of forces that the cells can apply. This is consistent with the fact that the layer loses actin stress fibres in the process of the layer getting denser (see chapter 4.1.3 and [190]) and has less space for lamellipodia and similar protrusions, that are associated with epithelial cell movement. It also corresponds well to the process of contact-inhibition of locomotion for epithelial-like cells, which is long known [259, 260, 241, 261, 262] and was for a while put forward as sole reason of an arrest in epithelial motion in densely-packed tissue, before the concept of jamming rose to prominence [263, 29]. This picture of slow-down in intrinsic cell movement corresponds well to the hypothesis formulated at the end of the last paragraph, where it was described that an environment high in cell number density is amplifying an underlying shape-induced jamming transition. There are of course other possible contributing factors to the influence of a high number density on the ability of cell rearrangements. For example, it has been shown recently by Han et al., that cell stiffness increases for the denser inside of spheroids, which the authors also correlated with lower cell velocities [264]. Since the moving cell and its local environment has to be remodelled during tissue rearrangement in a dense environment it seems clear that an increased cell stiffness is a hindrance to tissue rearrangement. At the moment there are no models that explicitly include these factors and all models known to me are scale invariant and have no easy way to include the cell number density. This includes an interesting new model of deformable polygons, which is able to reproduce the results of shape-dependent jamming of confluent layers in vertex models and expand it to scenarios with a volume fraction below one, combing the effect of cell shapes and holes in the tissue on the degrees of freedom of cells [47].

Is the tissue arrest jamming or glass-like?

Switching the topic of discussion to the description of the arrest in motion of cellular tissues as either glassy or jammed, which is admittedly slightly academic in some sense, as both concepts describe similar behaviour and are closely related. From a pedantic physical point of view the glassy terminology is the right one, as Berthier et al. outlined: "(...) jamming is understood as a purely geometric transition between viscous and rigid behavior in the absence of any kind of dynamics. Thus, jamming is a (...) zero-temperature and zero-activity limit. Strictly speaking, therefore, particles with nonvanishing activity cannot undergo jamming."[177] Nevertheless, the regimes of jammed and glassy behaviour share many similarities, and for a while, until it became clear that the Gardener (glass) transition and the jamming transition lead to differences, there was even a confusion among experts in the field whether or not these phenomena are the same at the core [265, 266, 193]. The difference between jamming and the Gardener transition to marginal glasses becomes apparent in theories of hard spheres in infinite dimensions by different scaling behaviours for contact forces and holes between spheres [193, 267, 268], but these are not appreciable in the complex systems of biological tissues. The terminology of jamming has a historic origin for biological systems as an influential theory was first developed for displacements of static cells and therefore coined the observed solidification jamming [30]. The other reason for the use of the term jamming is that it is easier to grasp, as even Berthier et al. admitted [177], which is extremely useful in interdisciplinary communication of physicists with biologist and physicians, who have no intuition what the term glass transition entails. The ease of communication is the main reason, that the term jamming is sticking for the arrest in motion within biological tissue, similar to the improbability of the scenario, that the general public will rename traffic jams into traffic glasses in order to match the correct physics terminology. This general tendency in the literature to use the term jamming is also the reason why I used it throughout this thesis.

Besides these considerations, there are intuitions attached to the terms glass and jamming, whose applicability on tissues I want to discuss. A glass transition implies a diverging viscosity controlled by a critical temperature, or in the case of self-propelled particles like cells a critical activity, that controls the transition between solid and fluid behaviour. In contrast, a jamming transition implies a critical volume fraction or cell shape, which can conceptually be united into a critical amount of degrees of freedom. It is clear that the yield-stress of jammed tissue could always be overcome by cell activity, if it is high enough. The activity of cells, which is sometimes coined intrinsic velocity, requires the exertion of forces by cells, which are limited by the amount of motor proteins, force transmitting cytoskeleton proteins and the adhesion strength of the cell, which can all be regulated by cells but only to a certain extend. Therefore, there are physiological boundaries on the activity of cells. The practical relevant question is, whether it is more useful to simplify the arrest of cellular motion as a transition depending on the internal activity or as a transition defined by the degrees of freedom available.

The intrinsic velocity of cells can not be easily measured in cells. An interesting future approach to investigate this problem would be a combination of traction force microscopy and cell jamming analysis. Currently, the clearest argument against a purely activity driven transition is the behaviour of arrested epithelial-like cell layers, when the boundary conditions change. If there is suddenly free space, the cells can start to move and, for example, close a wound. In doing so they move collectivity and exhibit very long correlation lengths [195, 269, 22, 94], that resemble the diverging cluster sizes near a glass or jamming transition [270, 271, 272, 273]. Importantly, as I discussed in figure 4.6, the amount of rearrangements within the layer does not necessarily increase during the wound healing process. This means that the cells are still caged by their neighbours and have to move coordinated with them. These cells are still jammed by their neighbours at a local level even though their intrinsic cell velocity is still high enough for fast collective motion, and they can close wounds at roughly the speed of individual cells [22]. These considerations are not totally new, as the phenomenon of flocking is known for epithelial cells and is even connected to jamming with a transition of jamming to solid flocks for an increasing cell alignment [195, 186, 94, 187]. At least from my point of view, this is currently not considered strongly enough, as a significant percentage of the literature does not consider relative cell motion and equates an increasing absolute amount of cell motion with unjamming, even if it is a strongly correlated motion of very large clusters and therefore still very close to the jamming transition [26, 188, 178]. This means that the ability of cells to rearrange is best described by the degrees of freedom available and is only modified by potential increases or reductions in the internal activity.

An example of the of such a modification by changes in the cell activity is the hypothesis I introduced in the previous chapter, which states that the cell number density reduces the intrinsic velocity and thereby increases the effect of the shape-dependent jamming. Furthermore, there are reports that RAB5A, an endocytic protein, can lead to unjamming of epithelial layers, by increasing traction and protrusions which are correlated with the cell velocity [185, 186, 187, 188]. The cell movement reported for alterations with RAB5A is always strongly correlated [185, 186, 187, 188], which resembles the diverging dynamic correlation length near a glass transition and therefore indicates that the system is not far from an arrest of motion, even if the overall velocity of cells might be high. There was an increase in the cell shape in these experiments and a decrease in adhesion via an increase in the turnover of molecules responsible for cell junctions [185, 188, 189]. Nevertheless, these experiments still indicate that an unjamming through increased cell activity can occur in nature. This could be described well as a glass-like phenomenon, but it still is an exception and the systems that I studied are relatively independent of the intrinsic velocity and are therefore well described by the framework of jamming.

The degrees of freedom of cells in tissues, estimated through cell shapes and volume fractions have turned out to be a reliable predictor of the state of motility in the tissue. In all of the three experimental systems presented in this work, the cell shape of fluid-like tissues was reliably higher than the ones of solid-like tissue, even if the solid-like tissue was not completely arrested. This is reflected in the literature, where the cell shape and volume fraction have proven to be good indicators of cell jamming in many cases in the literature [26, 164, 163, 185, 179, 53, 178]. There has been no reported case of fluid-like cell behaviour of a confluent tissue with round cells. In summary, a jamming transition of cells, defined by their degrees of freedom and modulated by their activity, describes my data best while being consistent with the literature. Hereby, the degrees of freedom correspond to the volume fraction of cells and their cell shapes while the cell activity can be modulated by biological cues like RAB5A [185, 188] as well as the physical cell environment, such as the number density of close by cells or possibly the stiffness and stickiness of substrates. This means that the structure of tissues and especially the shapes of its constituting cells is the primary determining factor of the state of its motility.

Cell biological changes connected to jamming

In order to connect the jamming and unjamming transition of tissues to known biological processes it is crucial to investigate the biological changes that instantiate the physical transitions. This is necessary to develop predictive models of cancer progression and might also inspire cellular alterations that reverse unjamming. I studied the effect of cell-cell adhesion in two parts of this thesis. The data shown in chapter 4.2, that were produced in a collaboration with the group of Prof. Friedl and published in Nature Cell Biology, showed that the down regulation of E-cadherin in a cancer cell line that has retained epithelial characteristics can individualise the cells and increase both their cell shape and fluidity [33]. On the surface, this is at odds with the currently prevalent theories of cellular jamming, that connect a decrease in adhesion with a decrease in surface energy of the cells, rounder cell shapes and would predict a higher likelihood of the system being jammed [30, 31, 32]. One fact that complicates the situation is, that a down-regulation of E-cadherin can have a cascading effect on other cell properties such as cortical contractility and traction [231, 232, 38, 34, 274]. Nevertheless, my data shows that a strong enough loss of adhesion can disrupt the cohesion of the of tissue, thereby introduce holes and decrease the volume fraction, which leads to an increase in the degrees of freedom of cells and their motility. The dependency of cell shape on adhesion is not a prediction of the SPV model of cell jamming, but a heuristic motivation of the used Hamiltonian [30, 32]. Nevertheless, the observed switch to a tissue of lower volume fraction motivates the development and refinement of models that can describe these, like the one proposed by Boromand et al. [47]. Switching the experimental system, I did not observe a striking change in the amount and structure of E-cadherin and desmosome molecules during the solidification of the MCF-10A layers I observed in chapter 4.1.3. This means that an increase in friction through adhesion is not necessary for jamming, contrary to an early hypothesis [27]. In summary, cell jamming requires a high amount of cell-cell adhesion to ensure a cohesive tissue at a high volume fraction, but is not driven primarily by adhesion.

The primary change visible between early confluence and a jammed-like state in the fluorescently labelled structure of cells was the restructuring of the actin cytoskeleton (see chapter 4.1.3). In contrast to earlier stages, there are no actin stress fibres visible in the cytoskeleton of layers close to a dynamic arrest and the actin is concentrated in cortex structures. This is in agreement to recent publications, which state that a change in traction through stress fibre contractility coincides with the jamming transition in their system [190], as well as experiments that induced an unjamming in nearly jammed cell layers via RAB5A, which biophysically mainly increases traction [185]. Conceptually, the effect of vanishing stress fibres is two-fold: Since these structures are used in cell motion, their disappearance presumable coincides with a reduced cell activity. Additionally, stress fibres tend to polarise cells increasing the cell shapes in the system. From a coarse-grained perspective this change can be understood as a transition from an inherently asymmetric stress fibre structure to a more symmetric cortex pattern. This changes the stresses that cells tend to evoke from an anisotropic profile, that is connected to motility and allows for many degrees of freedom on a tissue level to an isotropic profile on the level of cells connected to a lower intrinsic velocity, rounder cells and less degrees of freedom on a tissue level. Overall, this data indicates that a change in the structure of the actin cytoskeleton, via contractility of myosin II, is the primary biophysical change responsible for jamming and unjamming in confluent tissue.

An additional cell property, that might be important for rearrangements in densely-packed tissue, and is currently not considered in this context, is the stiffness of nuclei. This property has been studied in the context of cell migration through the extracellular matrix and narrow constrictions but not in the context of cell jamming [48, 49, 50, 58, 59, 60, 61]. Observing the cell rearrangements in fluid-like MDA-MB-436 spheroids, as showcased in figure 4.34b, one becomes aware that the nuclei are often strongly deformed during the rearrangements. This deformation has to require energy and therefore should be considered in a Hamiltonian of cell motion in dense tissue. Currently, the nucleus is not considered either directly nor indirectly in theories of cell jamming. This is a possible explanation why theories tend to underestimate the critical shape of cell jamming, such as in my data of three-dimensional spheroids shown in figure 4.37. These considerations are validated with the observations that the cell shapes and nucleus shapes are highly correlated in these spheroids (see figure 4.40) and that nuclei shapes correlate with the mobility of cells in time series of primary tumour pieces, where the cell shapes are hard to determine (see figure 4.44). Combined, this is strong evidence that the deformation of the nucleus required for cell rearrangements contributes to the energy barrier for cell rearrangements in jammed tissues. This shows that the considerations of nucleus deformability in studies of single cell movement is transferable to densely-packed tissues and the nucleus shape and stiffness is an important influence on cell jamming that is not considered until now.

Relevance for cancer

I will end this thesis with a discussion of the relevance of its content for cancer and give a short outlook of future research in this direction suggested by this thesis. Together with a recent preprint [181], the data presented in chapter 4.2 and published in Nature Cell Biology [33] shows for the first time, that the down-regulation of E-cadherin, a hallmark of the epithelial-mesenchymal transition connected with cancer development, can fluidise spheroids of cancer cells. This data was produced *in vitro* and confirmed with *in vivo* experiments in mice. The cells used in my work on this project where cells of the 4T1 cancer cell line, that is classified as metastatic but still retains epithelial characteristics, like the expression of E-cadherin [43, 44]. The observed fluidisation for the E-cadherin down regulated phenotype manifests itself as cell individualisation and a loss of persistence and spatial correlation of motion. The E-cadherin down regulated cells can move freely without coordinating with their neighbours, while cells of the original 4T1 cell type move in clusters, which had a low relative cell motion towards each other. This leads the E-cadherin high cell phenotype to move collectively and persistent, which is efficient in the absence of obstacles, illustrated by a super-diffusive exponent of the mean squared displacement. However, only the E-cadherin low phenotype can individualise and invade the boundary of collagen with individual cells. This behaviour is also consistent between *in vitro* and *in vivo* experiments, but can be blocked by a collagen networks, that are dense enough.

The preprint mentioned above studies an epithelial system in two dimensions and induces an unjamming transition either by mechanical compression or by triggering a partial epithelial-mesenchymal transition using TGF-β1 which is comparable to the down regulation of E-cadherin in my work [181]. They find that the unjamming transition caused by mechanical compression exhibits collective motion of large clusters, while the motion that is induced by a partial epithelial-mesenchymal transition is much less correlated [181]. In the framework that I am presenting, this means that the compression only shifts the system slightly past the jamming transition, since most cells are still locally caged by their neighbours, while the partial epithelial-mesenchymal transition induces a robust fluid behaviour, which is very consistent with the data I am presenting.

Overall this means that during full or partial epithelial-mesenchymal transition the E-cadherin loss, and subsequent changes of cell properties, initiates an unjamming transition. The behaviour of E-cadherin high cells is locally caged, leading to a state at least close to jamming for strong boundary condition and collective, persistent motion into regions that offer less resistance. The down regulation of E-cadherin leads to a fluid like state, where cells can move quite freely past their neighbours and move in a diffusive pattern if no other cues, like a path of least resistance, are present. Cancer cells in this low E-cadherin state can individualise and, for example, invade boundaries of sufficiently permeable extracellular matrix on their own. This means that the physical process of unjamming is connected to the biological process of the epithelial-mesenchymal transition, which is a hallmark of cancer progression and induces changes in the invasion behaviour of tumours.

Other experiments in the publication showed that fluid-like cells can also be funnelled into a path of least resistance by their environment even though their motion is presumable still fluid-like since the density of collagen boundaries did not change the qualitative cell motion in the experiments I analysed [33]. These paths of least resistance are similar to previously observed motion of cancer cells along tissue interfaces that have been described as collective motion [89, 100]. This means that not all observed movement that has been described as collective by biologists has to have large correlation lengths of cell velocities and thereby behave collectively in the terminology that physicists use. Which mode of motility is more efficient in cancer metastasis is not a priori clear and experiments in mice found no significant difference between the ability to metastasise between E-cadherin high and low 4T1 cells [33]. Presumably the collective persistent motion of E-cadherin high cells is more efficient in situations where the local environment provides less resistance, like in tissue interfaces or ducts, and individual cells can overcome obstacles that are not permeable for a group of cells sticking together. This leads to the hypothesis that the state of motility of the tumour, together with the properties of the local environment, have predictive power regarding the danger of metastasis and I could imagine that future studies find that different fluidities of the tumour allow for different target regions of metastasis, thereby helping to achieve a more focused and individualised detection and treatment of cancer. The often cited tumour heterogeneity can of course also influence this behaviour and potentially allow tumours to pursue different invasion strategies at the same time. These findings are part of a current shift in dogma from regarding the epithelial-mesenchymal transition as necessary for tumour invasion [34] to a modulating factor of metastasis [161, 155]. Of course motility is only one important step required for cancer metastasis, besides for example a resistance to the immune system [34, 275, 276, 277], but importantly this line of inquiry gives orthogonal and therefore truly new information, besides the currently modern genetic and biochemical approach.

Furthermore, I showed for the first time that the jamming and unjamming of confluent three-dimensional tissue is connected with the cell and nucleus shape (see chapter 4.4). While the connection with the cell shape was at least qualitatively predicted by theories [32, 46], there were no previous discussions of a connection between the state of motility in confluent tissue and the shapes of the cell nuclei involved, even though it appears to be an obvious possibility in hindsight as this connection was thoroughly discussed for individual moving cells in the presence of obstacles [48, 49, 50, 58, 59, 60, 61]. Importantly, the dependency of cell motion and nucleus shape could be confirmed for primary tumour pieces, which typically behaved jammed at least in some parts and frequently had unjammed regions of uncoordinately moving cells (see chapter 4.4.3). As discussed previously, this is evidence that the nucleus deformations required for cell rearrangements in densely packed tissue contribute to the energy barriers in jammed systems. This renders the nucleus stiffness a potentially important parameter for cell jamming and it is interesting to note that cancer cells typically have a reduced nuclei stiffness [278, 279]. There was no sequential change in the characteristics of the tumour pieces compared to their clinical grading discernible. Even tumour pieces at lower stages could contain fluid regions. However, the samples between different patients showed partially different behaviours raising the hope that one might be able to correlate these differences with patient outcome in the future. All the structural parameters like cell shape, cell number density, volume fraction and nucleus shape can be estimated in histological slides that are the standard tool for cancer diagnosis. Therefore, the findings in this thesis describe a framework that is able to predict the dynamical behaviour of tissues using their structure. This is an excellent starting point for the development of a hypothesis-driven predictive marker of cancer metastasis, which is described in more detail in the outlook. It is important to note that the here described kind of fluidisation through cell motility dominates over proposed processes of fluidisation through cell division in tumours [211, 212, 280], as breast tumours have a median doubling time of 150 days with large variations [281, 282, 283] and the typical time that fluid cells need to move a cell size in the fluid regions of my data is 4 hours.

Chapter 6

Outlook

My thesis contains strong evidence for a shape-dependent jamming transition in confluent tissue. It also shows that an unjamming occurs when the volume fraction of cells decreases drastically. Thereby, my data combines the theories of shape-dependent and density-dependent jamming that are often considered to describe the same transition with different assumptions [28, 32]. My data suggests that they instead describe different aspects of the same transition and a jammed solid-like state requires both a very high volume fraction of cells and round cell shapes. This provides a justification for the existence of both kinds of theories in parallel, explains why there were seemingly contradicting experimental findings and is fundamental for models trying to combine both effects.

Besides the density effect of the volume fraction that is analogue to the control parameter used for jamming in granular materials, I observed an influence of the cell number density on the cell jamming transition. The cell number density is currently not considered in models of cell jamming, which are typically scale free. While the effect of the cell number density seems to be consistent with a reduced internal velocity, this is an aspect where current models of cell jamming could be improved. Another possibility is that the influence of the cell number density could be connected to the effect of required nuclei deformations for cell rearrangements, which is also not considered in models of cell jamming. A higher cell number density potentially increases the deformations of the nuclei necessary for cell rearrangements thereby increasingly contributing to the energy barrier for cell rearrangements in jammed tissue. The results of this thesis contribute to the understanding of cell jamming and different modes of unjamming. I hope that they will inspire improved models of this phenomenon.

My thesis also lays the foundations for future translational research. The central statement and common theme throughout this thesis is that the dynamical behaviour of tissues is reflected in their structure. This suggests the hypothesis that the structure of clinical samples can be analysed in order to draw conclusions about their dynamics and therefore potentially their hazard, which would be of great importance for the improvement of prognosis by histopathology. My thesis shows that especially the cellular and nuclear shape are strong predictors of the dynamic behaviour of cells in confluent tissue. The volume fraction of cells is another central parameter for cell jamming, which is not currently quantified in conventional pathological diagnosis. These parameters, together with modulating influences from, for example, the cell number density and properties of the extracellular matrix should be able to predict the motile state of cancer cells and thereby provide strong statements about the metastatic ability of individual tumours. These considerations together with the data presented in this thesis have triggered a cooperation of the group of my supervisor Prof. Käs with the pathologist Prof. Niendorf, whose aim and approach I will shortly illuminate in the following paragraphs.

The complexity of the disease and the invasiveness of its treatments render the grading of cancer and treatment decisions both important and hard, which leads to both over- and undertreatment of patients [284, 285]. This invokes a drastic cost on human life and well-being making potential improvements a high priority. The central pillar of cancer diagnosis is still pathological slides of suspicious tissue, that are graded by human pathologist, who mainly rely on long-standing empirical heuristics. This is not intrinsically wrong, but promises room for improvement. There is currently a large amount of research into machine learning approaches for grading pathological slides, which are promising in their own right [286, 287]. However, humans tend to be sceptical when asked to rely on black box algorithms for life altering decisions and maybe even have a point as negative examples like biased machine learning algorithms in court estimating the likelihood of relapsing into crime by skin colour and social standing show [288]. The orthogonal approach is to develop a sensible hypotheses, such as modelling the threat of cancer metastasis as a interaction between tissue fluidity and local environment and measuring estimator using histological slides. This could later be combined with genetic information of the cancer completing the picture. The best possible outcome to work towards to would be a predictive marker that can model the tumour and environment properties and predict the most likely future development of

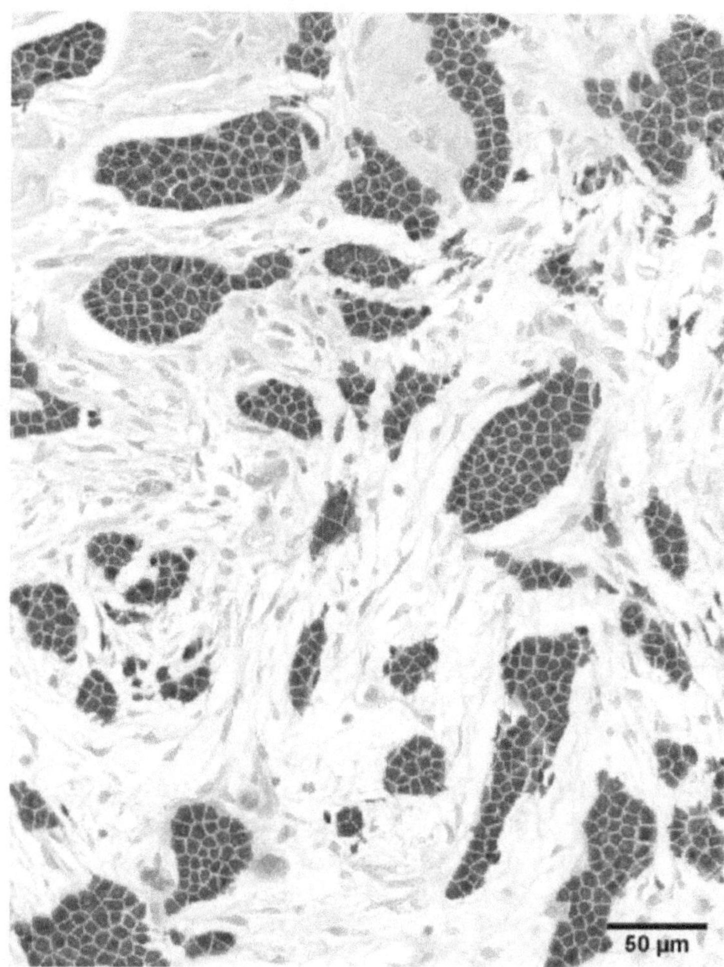

Figure 6.1: Histological slide of breast cancer with hematoxylin and eosin (HE) stain. Outlines of an automated nuclei detection are overlaid in red and a Voronoi-tesselation around the nuclei centres of cancer cells is overlaid in white. Figure by Pablo Gottheil, Jürgen Lippoldt, Josef A. Käs, Axel Niendorf.

the particular tumour, compared to the prognostic markers currently deployed that sort the patients into statistical classes of different dangerousness [289].

As indicated previously, the work on this project has already begun in a cooperation between the pathologist Prof. Niendorf and the group of my supervisor Prof. Käs. I guided a master student, Pablo Gottheil, who adapted my cell segmentation analysis, used in chapter 4.2.1 and 4.4.2, to histological slides and continues this project now as a PhD student. It has already been shown, that slices through three-dimensional tissue retain information about the three-dimensional structure [254]. Figure 6.1 shows an exemplary section of a histological slide with breast cancer, whose nuclei are segmented and marked with a red outline. The cell shapes of the cancerous cells in this image are estimated by a Voronoi-tesselation around the nuclei shown as an overlay of bright lines. The initial results of this project are very promising. A combined measure of cell shape, nucleus shape and their width of distributions, showed a statistical significant difference between patients that later developed metastasis and those who did not. This was done in an ensemble that was not separably for human pathologists, and coined 'grey zone' tissue microarray by Prof. Niendorf. The additional information this measure provides are therefore a good first step, which will be improved in the future by analysing more data and incorporating more information, like properties of the cancer environment for reasons described above. Interestingly, some of these structural variables, that were chosen because they are connected to the motility of the tissue, as described in this thesis, were already regarded as important by pathologists empirically. The nucleus shape and its variance is part of the criterion of pleomorphism already described in the 1950's and still used today [51, 52]. On the other hand, the cell shape is not an usual estimator, since it is not apparent in a slide stained with hematoxylin and eosin, but even if the Voronoi tesselation does only estimate and not fully capture the real cell shape, the information about the order of the tissue seems to be relevant, as both chapter 4.3 in my thesis and the initial data of this project demonstrate. In summary of this outlook, it is great to be able to state that my work has motivated and informed a project that will directly save lives if it pans out as we think it will.

Appendix A

Protocol appendix

A.1 Cell and spheroid culture

Media

MCF-10A cells were cultured in MCF-10A-medium:
DMEM/Ham's F12 medium with L-glutamine (Cat.No. E15-813, PAA Laboratories GmbH, Austria) supplemented with 5% horse serum (Cat.No. A15-151, PAA), $20\,\mathrm{ng\,l^{-1}}$ human EGF (Cat.No. E9644, Sigma-Aldrich), $10\,\mathrm{\mu g\,l^{-1}}$ insulin (Cat. No.I9278, Sigma-Aldrich), $100\,\mathrm{ng\,l^{-1}}$ cholera toxin (Cat.No. C8052, Sigma-Aldrich), $500\,\mathrm{ng\,l^{-1}}$ hydrocortisone (Cat.No. H0888, Sigma-Aldrich) and 100 U/ml penicillin/streptomycin (Cat.No. P11-010, PAA).

MDA-MB-436 cells were cultured in MDA-medium:
DMEM containing $4.5\,\mathrm{g\,l^{-1}}$ glucose, L -glutamine, but without sodium pyruvate (Cat.No. E15-810, PAA) supplemented with 10% fetal bovine serum (Cat.No. A15-151, PAA) and 100 U/ml penicillin/streptomycin.

All cell lines were incubated at 37°C in a 5% CO_2 atmosphere. The culture medium was changed every 2-3 days and cells were passaged every 4-5 days.

Cell passaging

To detach the cells, cells were rinsed twice with PBS to remove medium. A PBS solution containing 0.025%(w/v) trypsin and 0.01%(w/v) EDTA (Cat.No. L11-004, PAA) was applied for 15 min for MCF-10A, and 5 min for MDA-MB-436.

As soon as all cells have detached, threefold to fivefold amount of culture medium was added to inhibit trypsin using a serological pipette. Cells are centrifuged at 100 g for 4 min. The supernatant is removed and cells are resuspended in 1 ml fresh medium.

Spheroid culture

After passage, cells in the cell suspension were counted using a cell counter. The desired number of cells was pipetted in non-adherent 96-U-well plates (Cat.No 781900, BRAND), which had been filled with 100 µL medium.

Spheroids of both cell types were cultivated in 50/50 medium, a mixture of 50% of MCF-10A-medium and MDA-medium, to ensure that the observed features are cell-type dependent (thus not a mere consequence of medium formulation) and to achieve consistency with my previous publication on spheroid segregation [170].

Both cell types also grow well in 50/50 medium in flasks, and I have repeated key experiments of this work in the corresponding "pure" media. MCF-10A spheroids still show jammed characteristics in MCF-10A medium, while MDA-MB-436 spheroids also show the fluid characteristics in MDA medium (data not shown).

A.2   Acquisition of spheroid bulk fusion data

The same non-adherent 96-wells were filled with 150 µl of fresh medium, and a pair of spheroids was placed in each well: Spheroids were moved between wells using a 1 ml pipette tip, whose opening is much larger than the spheroids.

As a result, spheroids moved to the bottom of the wells, where they met within a few minutes to one hour.

Bright-field images of the fusion process are recorded using a Leica N PLAN 5X/0.12 objective every 5 min using a CCD camera at cell incubation conditions (37 °C,

$5\% \ CO_2$).

A.3 Tumour transport and preparation

The tissue is transported in a modified ringer tissue buffer based on Ringer's Lactate Solution. This buffer solution keeps the integrity of the tissue intact (just using phosphate buffer solution (PBS) does not contain sufficient chemical energy sources).

This procedure was based on a recommendation by the Biozentrum of the university of Basel. As basis for the Modified Ringer Tissue Buffer serves a Ringer's lactate solution (B. Braun Medical AG, Cat.No. 3325950, Approval No. 6724011.00.00) supplemented with 5% [w/v] glucose monohydrate and 1% Antibiotic-Antimycotic Solution (PAA, Cat.No. P11-002) to suppress possible contaminations.

Tumour pieces are then cut coarsely in a 100 mm dish filled with Dulbecco's Modified Eagle's Medium (DMEM).

A.4 Sample preparation and microscopy for live observation

A.4.1 Monolayers

For monolayers experiments, cells were seeded into 24-well plates with flat microscopy bottom (ibidi) at a cell density slightly below the desired starting density of the experiment. The well plates were incubated over night, to allow the cells to attach fully.

The time series was acquired on a ZEISS Axio Observer spinning disc microscope using a nuclear vital stain of (0.2 µM SiR-DNA, Spirochrome). The images were taken with a ZEISS EC Plan-Neofluar M27 10X/0.3 objective allowing large image sections. Multiple sections were recorded in parallel and each section was imaged once every 10 min over 3 days.

The experiment was conducted inside an incubation chamber with a large reservoir of medium. The deep-red ($\Lambda_{ex} = 638$ nm) illumination minimizes toxicity, as compared to smaller wavelengths. To ensure that the signal does not deteriorate during the observation time, spheroids are placed in medium supplied with 0.2 µM SiR-DNA, which is below the maximum concentration for live imaging recommended by the vendor of 1 µmol.

A.4.2   Spheroids and tissue pieces

For spheroids, 150-200 cells were grown for 1 day in 384-well plates with flat microscopy bottom (ibidi), coated with 17 µl of 1% agarose. This coating creates U-shaped wells, which however are thin enough to allow for high-NA imaging.

Tumours were cut into pieces using scalpels. Tumour pieces were transferred into the same wells and same medium as spheroids.

Images were acquired on a ZEISS Axio Observer spinning disc microscope. I recorded nuclear vital stain (0.2 µM SiR-DNA, Spirochrome) fluorescence signals every 5 or 7.5 min, for at least 6 h, sometimes up to 24 h.

The experiment was conducted inside an incubation chamber with a large reservoir of medium. The deep-red ($\Lambda_{ex} = 638$ nm) illumination minimizes toxicity and is superior in penetration depth, as compared to smaller wavelengths. The high-NA water immersion objective ZEISS C-Apochromat 40X/1.2W was used to achieve a good signal-to-noise ratio, and to match sample and immersion refractive indices. To ensure that the signal does not deteriorate during the observation time, spheroids are placed in medium supplied with 0.2 µM SiR-DNA, which is below the maximum concentration for live imaging recommended by the vendor of 1 µmol.

A.5   Sample preparation for fixation, staining, and 3D segmentation

Fixation and labelling of cell monolayers

For keratin/desmoplakin and actin/e-cadherin labelling of 2D cell layers, monolayers were prepared by fixating in cold methanol ($-20\,°C$) or 10% Formalin (Sigma-Aldrich, HT5011), respectively, for 15 minutes, and afterwards treated with 1% Triton™ X-100 solution (Sigma-Aldrich, 93443) and 5% BSA (Sigma-Aldrich, A2153-50G) in PBS.

For keratin and desmoplakin labelling, the monolayers were incubated for 1 hour at room temperature with anti-cytokeratin PAN rabbit polyclonal antibody (Thermo Fisher Scientifc, PA1-27114), and anti-desmolplakin mouse monoclonal antibody (L278) kindly donated by the Magin Lab (Institute of Biology, University of Leipzig). After intermediate washing steps, the layer was further incubated for 30 minutes with goat anti-rabbit IgG (H+L) highly cross-adsorbed secondary antibody, Alexa Fluor Plus 647 (Thermo Fisher Scientific, AB_2633282) and goat anti-mouse IgG (H+L) highly cross-adsorbed secondary antibody, Alexa Fluor 488 (Thermo Fisher Scientific, AB_2534088).

For actin and e-cadherin labelling the monolayers were incubated for 1 hour at room temperature with e-cadherin mouse monoclonal antibody (HEDC-1) (Thermo Fisher Scientific, AB_2533003), and then for 30 minutes with SiR-actin (Spirochrome, SC001), and with the previously mentioned goat anti-mouse IgG (H+L) highly cross-adsorbed secondary antibody, Alexa Fluor 488.

Hoechst-34580 (Molecular Probes, H21486) was added to the secondary antibody solution to label the nuclei.

Fixation and staining of spheroids and tumour pieces

Spheroids and tumour samples were fixed using 4% [w/v] paraformaldehyde in PBS for 30 min. This fixation time was chosen longer than for regular adhered cells, as PFA needs more time to penetrate into thicker tissue pieces.

Samples were then consecutively washed using PBS, transferred to a solution consisting of 1% Triton-X and 1% BSA for at least 2 h, better 24 h, then washed using PBS. Washing steps are done by letting spheroids sink to the ground of the wells and pipetting the supernatant to about 90% off, and then refilling with the respective liquid. Depending on the concentrations needed, this step hast to be repeated iteratively, i.e. to remove PFA from the samples as complete as possible.

Staining was done with 0.1 µM SiR-DNA (Spirochrome) for labeling DNA, and Alexa-Fluor 488 Phalloidin (Thermo-Fisher, Waltham), or Alexa-Fluor 532 Phalloidin, for about 24 h to label actin.

Optical clearing of spheroids and tumour pieces

For imaging, spheroids/samples were moved using a tilt 20 μL pipette tip into *ibidi μ-Slide 18 Wells (Flat)* (ibidi, Munich, Germany) with microscopy bottom. To help find the spheroids, this is done on a microscopy with a low-magnification objective (e.g. 4X).

The liquid quickly starts to evaporate, so the next step should be done soon afterwards. For optical clearing of the spheroids, *ibidi IMM* mounting medium was added. Its refractive index (RI) was measured using a refractometer: $n \approx 1.445$. This medium provides for sufficient optical clearing in spheroids up to about 200 μm size. As it is based on a glycerol-water mixture, it automatically adjusts to the atmospheric humidity, acquiring the aforementioned RI.

Optical clearing is very rapid and happens within seconds to minutes.

Confocal imaging of fixated spheroids and tumour pieces

Fluorescence images were acquired on Leica TCS SP2 and TCS SP5 confocal microscopes, using different objectives and immersion media. I have investigated how objective resolution, index mismatch between clearing and immersion medium, noise and other factors affect the results, and have devoted a section of the methods chapter to that information.

Most results were imaged using Leica HC PL APO 20X/0.7 CS Corr IMM objective with a glycerol/water mixture ($n = 1.45$) as immersion, avoiding any RI-mismatch between sample and immersion medium.

A.6 Optical stretcher measurements and analysis

Before the experiments cells were cultivated until they had the desired confluency and then were detached by trypsination and transferred into a single-cell suspension. The suspension is then injected into the microfludic system of the optical stretcher (RS Zelltechnik). Cells were first trapped by counter-propagating lasers, with an Gaussian laser profile, with a laser power 100 mW each. After one second increased the laser power to 875 mW, forcing the deformation of the trapped cell. This increased the temperature of the cell to 37°C. The cell deformation was recorded for 5 seconds. After the 5 seconds, the laser power was reduced to 100mW to keep the cell stable. The relaxation of the cell was observed for another two seconds. This process is done automated for each cell individually.

The analysis of the measurement is based on the deformations on the cell shape, which is automatically evaluated by an edge detection. The actin cortex contractility was estimated with an extended active Kelvin-Voight model [205, 206].

$$\epsilon(t) = \frac{1}{E}\left[(\sigma_{ext}) - \sigma_{int}^2 \cdot t + \Delta\sigma_{int}^2 \cdot \tau) - (\sigma_{ext}) + \Delta\sigma_{int}^2 \cdot \tau)\exp(\frac{-t}{\tau})\right] + \frac{\sigma_{ext} - \Delta\sigma_{int}^2 \cdot \tau}{E_2}$$

$$(A.1)$$

Thereby, σ_{ext} is the optical stress acting on the cell surface upon an optical laser power, $\Delta\sigma_{int}^2$ is the rate of cortical contractility of suspended cells, σ_{int}^2 is the total contractile stress after a 5 second stretch, $\epsilon(t)$ represents cell deformation upon external stress and potentially induced internal σ_{ext} contractile stress σ_{int}, E is the Elasticity of the suspended cells and E_2 an additional serial aligned elastic modulus.